Letters of Consequence

1912–2012
A History of the
Institute of Biomedical Science

Letters of Consequence

1912–2012
A History of the
Institute of Biomedical Science

David Petts and Tony Harding

Edited by Brian Nation

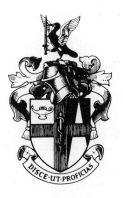

Institute of Biomedical Science

Published by the Institute of Biomedical Science
12 Coldbath Square, London EC1R 5HL, UK
Tel: +44 (0)20 7713 0214
Fax: +44 (0)20 7837 9658
Web: www.ibms.org

British Library Cataloguing in Publication Data
A catalogue record for this book is available from the British Library

ISBN 978-0-9570866-1-6

Distribution:
Institute of Biomedical Science
12 Coldbath Square, London EC1R 5HL, UK
Tel: +44 (0)20 7713 0214
Fax: +44 (0)20 7837 9658

Designed, typeset and printed by Berrington Press, Unit 1, Cae Brane, Rowlestone,
Pontrilas, Herefordshire HR2 0DL
Bound by Skyline Bookbinders

Preface

This is the third book to attempt to recount the history of the Institute of Biomedical Science (IBMS). The first, entitled *A Survey*, by W A (Walter) Mitchell told the story of the first 21 years (1912–1933) of the Pathological and Bacteriological Laboratory Assistants' Association (PBLAA). In 1982, Dr A D Farr published his important account of the history of the PBLAA and the first 40 years of the Institute, taking its title from the professional body's motto, 'Learn, that you may improve' (*Disce ut proficias*).

Other accounts have been proposed. In 1949 and 1950, G Harper proposed that the history from 1933 be written, but, on the advice of Albert Norman, this was deferred. In 1959, Council discussed the production of a history to coincide with the Institute's Golden Jubilee in 1962. It was thought that Albert Norman was most suited to write this and that a grant may be approved in order for him to take one month's leave from work to undertake the task. Again, this was not undertaken and, given our experience, it is very unlikely that a month would have been sufficient time, even for Albert Norman, well versed as he was in the Institute's affairs, to produce such a document.

In compiling the current account, we have drawn both inspiration and information from these earlier works and occasionally have quoted from them. Derek Farr, perhaps somewhat boldly, subtitled his book 'The History of the Institute of Medical Laboratory Sciences'; we, however, make no such claim – this is a history. It is our take on the development and activities of our professional body and attempts to give an account of what it has tried to achieve, and often succeeded in achieving, for its members and their profession. It is not intended to be an encyclopaedic history as neither time nor space would allow this.

Our hope is that we have been able to show how the ideals of John McLean and Albert Norman have been built upon and remain central to those of the IBMS. We also hope that we have shown how the relatively small PBLAA has grown and developed into a large, complex body with an outstanding international reputation, and how it influenced the development of the profession worldwide. With a membership that has risen from around 100 in 1912 to over 20,000 at the beginning of 2011, it has moved on from an exclusively male membership to one that is just over 60% female; from one with no formal educational requirements to one where to enter its corporate membership requires an accredited honours degree; and where postgraduate qualifications are necessary for upward progression through the classes of membership; and from one overseen, and in the early years given legitimacy, by the medical profession, to a self-regulating, independent professional body of national and international standing.

To produce this account we have relied heavily on the archives of the Institute and the memories of its senior members, both active and retired. The archives contain a complete set of *The Laboratory Journal* and its successor titles, *The Bulletin* and *The Gazette* (now *The Biomedical Scientist*), and the minute books of the PBLAA and Council, and some other committee minutes. Regrettably, probably as the result of several changes of premises, a lack of space and perhaps an occasional lack of appreciation of their historical value, many documents have been lost. This is particularly true of correspondence, and, because of this, the background discussion to proposals and decisions was often unavailable to us. As a result, our account of events may make them appear to have had a smoother passage than was the case in reality. Judging by some of the letters published in *The Gazette*, many developments were not universally popular. Fortunately, some very important letters have survived that had significant consequences for the Institute and its members. These, together with the post-nominal letters of professional qualifications (ie FIBMS, CSci), are the *Letters of Consequence* of the title.

In this account, wherever possible, we have steered away from producing a history of pathology and the development of methods and their myriad uses. Inevitably, the expansion of the science and the size and complexity of laboratories, and their importance to healthcare, has driven and informed the development of the Institute. Occasionally, these developments have brought the role of the Institute and its members under professional and political scrutiny, even under attack. However, over the past century, the Institute has endeavoured to maintain good relationships with the other professions, trades unions and governmental organisations to ensure that the development and status of its members is recognised. It has also reached out to provide assistance and support to nascent organisations that represent other careers related to pathology.

History is, of course, an account of things and events that have happened, but, inevitably, as the Institute continues into its second century, events continue to unfold as we write. We have alluded to some of these, but it is not possible to recount, or understand, their relevance to history until the dust has settled.

We hope that this account will at least give the reader an insight into the events which led to the development and rise of the Institute, and an appreciation of the men and women whose imagination, insight, hard work and dedication over the past century have steered its undoubted success as the premier professional body in its field.

David Petts
Tony Harding
Brian Nation

This work is dedicated to our respective families, specifically Pam, Brenda and Kim, in recognition of their help, understanding and forbearance, without which this enormous project could not have been completed.

Acknowledgements

We were both somewhat surprised when we were asked by Alan Potter to write a book on the history of the Institute of Biomedical Science to mark its centenary in 2012. After some thought, and with more than a little trepidation, we agreed. There were more than a few times when we wondered what we had let ourselves in for and whether we had accepted a 'poisoned chalice'.

No work of this nature can be written without the considerable help, advice and patience of others. There are many people whose help we gratefully acknowledge, and the order in which they are recorded here in no way ranks the degree of importance or the value of their contribution.

***

While the vast majority of our information was drawn from IBMS documents, several people provided or assisted us to find information in other libraries and archives. We are particularly grateful to the staff of the Centre for Research Collections at the Edinburgh University Library, and to Estela Dukan at the Royal College of Physicians of Edinburgh (RCPE) Library for the invaluable assistance in helping us find information on the early days of pathology in that city. Invaluable data were also received from Dr Thomas Gillespie of Wishaw Hospital.

Captain (Retd) Peter Starling, the curator of the Army Medical Services Museum in Aldershot, provided valuable information on the training of Army laboratory staff in the early 20th century. We would not have been able to calculate the probable number of British pathology laboratories in existence in 1912 without the help of Rosalind Pitts of the Pathological Society of Great Britain and Ireland (Path Soc), who found the list of members for 1910/11. Sorting out the information about the development of the Institute's examinations would have been much harder without the help of Dr Ray Jones, whose DPhil thesis *The Development of the Medical Laboratory Scientific Officer: Qualifying Systems, Professional Politics and Technical Change*, at the University of Sussex, was invaluable, as was his information about St David's Hospital, Carmarthen.

The more recent examinations and qualification systems were patiently and diligently explained to us by Alan Wainwright, the Institute's Executive Head of Education. This, together with the papers and documents, helped one of us (DNP), brought up in the 'old system', to get his head around the current system. The documents provided by Nigel Mobey and Dr Doreen King were also very helpful. The background details to the transition from Triennial conference to Congress, given by Robert Kyte of Step, were most illuminating and we are very grateful for his assistance with aspect of our history. John Foster, whose knowledge of the arrangements for the later Triennials and Congress is probably unparalleled, gave us very valuable information and documents relating to these important events. The details of the relationship between the Institute and CPA (UK) and the development of the accreditation system, provided by Cheryl Blair, were also very helpful.

***

It was particularly pleasing to discover how many colleagues from organisations outside the UK were both willing and able to help us in our search for information about their early years and contacts with both the Pathological and Bacteriological Laboratory Assistants' Association (PBLAA) and the Institute. Ian Stranger sent us some useful material about the early years in Australia. Similarly, Christine Nielsen of the Canadian Society for Medical Laboratory Science and Fran van Til of the New Zealand Institute of Medical Laboratory Science were very helpful. The information and support given by Tom Moloney of the Academy of Medical Laboratory Science in Ireland was greatly appreciated. Our thanks also go to His Excellency Joseph Tomusange, Ugandan Ambassador to Denmark and a former Fellow of the Institute, and to Ayika Ponsiano, for assisting us with information about the situation in Uganda and East Africa generally. Unfortunately, not all those outside the UK were able to help but we are nevertheless grateful for their interest in this project. Although not overseas, the organisation of the health services in Scotland and Northern Ireland differs from that in England, and Derek Bishop and Gordon McNair were able to give us an insight into the relationship between the IBMS and their respective administrations.

We were fortunate to have access the memories of two long-serving General Secretary/Chief Executives. We are extremely grateful to John Fawcett for his continuing interest in this book and the loan of personal and often unique documents. One of us (AJH) also had some very informative conversations with John. As we have already said, Alan Potter asked us to undertake this project and we are very grateful for his trust and confidence in our ability to undertake the task Alan also ensured that the administrative support we needed was available, and provided us with much valuable information on his time in office.

Several former Presidents were more than generous with their time and knowledge, and we are very grateful to (in alphabetical order) Jim Cloke, Jocelyn Craig (Germain), Martin Nicholson, Kenny Rae and Graham Smart.

Sadly, two extremely helpful gentlemen died during the writing of the book and we gratefully acknowledge the unstinting interest, support and help given to us by Tom Lansley and John Mercer. Tom's memory of events was remarkable and the conversations we enjoyed, plus the papers he wrote for us, all unbidden, on various aspects of the past, gave us very valuable background to events that we would otherwise only known about from minutes and edited reports. John, both in his role as the Institute's Librarian and as an historian, assisted us greatly with archived documents and books. Without him we would not have had a set of the Institute's Annual Reports to consult – they were his collection; the Institute did not have a set of its own. Both gentlemen are sadly missed and we regret that they will not see the fruits of our labours.

***

Inevitably, the research for this book involved spending many days in the Institute's office and the staff were very patient and helped us find information and extract data. Peter Smith was able to find background and briefing paper on a whole range of topics, and his memory of how things happened was a great help. Conversations with Hedley Glencross, Steven Johnson, Alice Madziwa and Christian Burt helped clarify our thoughts and provided many useful insights. Having eventually found an office on the first floor in which we could work, our grateful thanks go to the team of Joanna Budzowska-Gawlak, Edyta Koziarska, Karim Bhawan, Natalie Killiansmith and Rehan Begum, who dealt with interruptions and requests for help with great patience and forbearance. Nadine Rulliere and Julie Turner helped us greatly with various administrative and accommodation problems and this helped smooth our task. We must also express our gratitude to members of the IBMS History Committee who have not already been mentioned, Hilda Taylor, Stephen Clarke and John Bushrod, for their interest and support. Thanks also go to Alex Cochrane for information on the introduction and development of electronic communication with the membership, and to Jamie Ansell for help with the scanning of images.

Not all was plain sailing and without the help of the Deputy Chief Executive, Sarah May, the Chief Executive, Jill Rodney, and the President, Kenny Rae, to help us deal with some last-minute hiccups, the final stages of the production of this book would have been more fraught, and we are grateful for their help in resolving these difficulties.

***

A book written by people living several hundred miles apart, even with modern communications technology, is not straightforward and our special thanks must go to our editor, Brian Nation. He not only set out a framework against which we could work, but managed to harmonise our writing, meld our different styles, and when, on occasion, we had written on the same topic, ensured that we did not get boringly repetitive; all with good grace and a sense of humour. For all this, and the introductory scene setting at the beginning of each chapter, we are most grateful. As we draw to a close, mention should also be made of the unswerving help, support and cooperation provided by our designer and printer, Mark Jenner and David Wood, at Berrington Press, and also our proof-reader Lynne Trattles.

***

Our wives have been extremely patient while we have been engaged on this task and for this and their unswerving support we are more than grateful. Their help went further than just moral support – Brenda Harding undertook research at the National Archive and RCPE, while Pam Petts not only read and helped correct our draft manuscripts but also, after a great deal thought and discussions with David, suggested the title *Letters of Consequence*. For all of this and so much more, thank you.

David Petts
Tony Harding

Contents

Chapter 1

The Nineteenth Century

Pathology in Historical Context
Rise of the Founding Fathers

*Burke's the butcher, Hare's the thief, Knox, the man who buys the beef.
So goes the children's song that alludes to the way the demand for medical
knowledge through human dissection was satisfied in Edinburgh in the 1820s.
Another son of the Scottish capital, one Arthur Conan Doyle, who studied
medicine at the University of Edinburgh, devised the first meeting of Sherlock
Holmes and Dr Watson to take place in a laboratory at St Bartholomew's
Hospital in London. Medical science has been, and so remains, fertile ground
for those with imagination.*

Towards the end of the 19th century the leading centres of medical practice and research were Cambridge, Edinburgh, London, Oxford and Manchester. It can be argued that, with its many eminent physicians and surgeons practising at the forefront of research in their respective fields, Edinburgh led the field in research related to pathology. The earliest laboratory was established in the Department of Surgery in this city's Medical School by Professor John Chiene in 1884. It was created for research into, and teaching of, bacteriology. Its foundation was probably due, in no small part, to the interest and work of Joseph (later Lord) Lister, who returned to Edinburgh in 1870 and was greatly influenced by the work of Louis Pasteur.

In 1885, undoubtedly galvanised by the visit of Louis Pasteur to Edinburgh in the previous year, the Council of the Royal College of Physicians of Edinburgh (RCPE) commissioned a new medical laboratory for research, and this opened in 1887. This was much heralded by physicians and surgeons eager to carry out research in bacteriology, anatomy and physiology. Once the laboratory was established, it was realised that the medical personnel would need assistance and the laboratories would require cleaning, maintenance and supervision to keep them operational. To this end, the superintendent and the board of the laboratory set out to recruit men and boys to carry out these tasks.

The records of the RCPE laboratory show in detail those individuals who were recruited, and among this number were several men who were instrumental in forming the first assistants' association. These included John McLean and William Watson.

***

The pathology service in Edinburgh in 1896, when John McLean first tried to form a laboratory assistants' association, was rudimentary compared with the sophisticated service available to medical practitioners practising in the early years of the 21st century. Indeed, in Great Britain, clinical pathology laboratories were a relatively recent development and very few had been established.

Outside medical school departments, the primary function of which was teaching and research, up until the 1880s the scientific investigation of post-mortem and ante-mortem samples from patients was normally undertaken by individual physicians or surgeons, for the benefit of their own patients or for their own research interests. Specimens were rarely, if ever, referred to another doctor for opinion. Investigations were either carried out in the doctor's rooms or by junior staff or students in ward side rooms.

Consultants directed most effort to their private practice and the care of patients in hospital wards, whereas the governors of charitable hospitals had a duty to care for the poor and needy. So, neither group saw it as their role to provide laboratory services, and therefore, well into the 19th century, pathology in the UK primarily remained confined to the study of morbid anatomy, either during autopsies, often performed by students, or from museum specimens.

In the 17th century, students and surgeons used cadavers both as a source of learning and of discovery. However, the eminent anatomist William Harvey believed that more could be learned from the dissection of one man who had died of disease than from 10 hanged men. There are records showing that students at St Thomas' Hospital undertook these dissections and recorded their findings. Similarly, a surgeon at the same hospital gave the earliest description of cirrhosis of the liver in an alcoholic soldier on whom he had performed an autopsy.

By the early 19th century, most physicians and surgeons learned a great deal of their trade in the post-mortem room. When Guy's Hospital Medical School opened, in 1826, the study of pathology was an important part of the medical student's course of study. Although museum specimens played a major role in the teaching of pathology, these were normally the private property of the lecturer, not the medical school. To overcome this difficulty, doctors were often appointed as museum curators and demonstrators and were required to undertake the time-consuming work of obtaining and preparing specimens for the medical school museum. However, these appointments were often only of a part-time nature and were seen as a stepping stone to other posts.

Although medical schools appointed professors of pathology these men did not earn their living from these posts and could not be considered as professional pathologists. Some held more than one professorial chair at a time and again often used the post as a stepping stone to more remunerative clinical appointments.

Outside the formal teaching establishments, doctors formed societies which included the study of pathology in their aims. One such was the Belfast Clinical and Pathological Society. Formed in 1853, it had among its aims "the cultivation of practical pathology, diagnosis and therapeutics and the establishment of a pathological museum".

***

The observation of changes to the organs and bodily fluids as a result of disease has been part of medicine from the very earliest times. Hippocrates observed that there were variations in the colour and clarity of urine and that these changes were often associated with disease. Early writings described haematuria and pyuria, and Indian physicians around 500 AD observed that the urine of 'diabetics' was sweet.

In the 18th century there was an expansion of analytical chemistry, and physicians with an interest in this subject turned their attention to urine in order to determine its normal and abnormal constituents. During the latter part of the century, urea and uric acid were discovered, and in 1776 Mathew Dobson, a Liverpool physician, noted that diabetic urine underwent fermentation and that the residue formed after evaporation tasted of sugar.

Richard Bright showed that albumin was present in the urine of patients with nephritis and he tested for it by heating the urine in a spoon. Furthermore, examination of the appearance and condition of a patient's stool samples was considered of great importance by many 18th-century physicians.

Patients were often bled to improve the balance of their 'humours'. Although early phlebotomists recognised that there were sometimes differences in the amount of clot, 'buffy coat' and serum, the chemical and haematological changes of the blood were not investigated. In the 17th century, Robert Boyle investigated blood and John Locke demonstrated the presence of 'sea salt' in blood using silver nitrate. However, it was not really until the 19th century that the chemical and cellular properties of blood and the factors influencing coagulation began to be investigated. It was during this century that the significance of changes in the chemical and cellular constituents of blood in health, and in specific diseases, started to be recognised. For instance, in 1829 Chritison was able show that urea was raised in the blood and lowered in urine in chronic nephritis. In 1848, Garrod reported raised uric acid levels in patients with gout, and was able to show that gout and rheumatoid arthritis were different conditions.

Platelets were first described by Donné, and Gabriel Andral wrote, in 1844, an essay on pathological haematology and, in 1845, Virchow, Bennett and Donné all noted that the number of white cells was raised in leukaemia. Andral also discovered that red cells were reduced in anaemia; he did this by drying and weighing the cells. However, the first report of a red cell count did not appear until 1852 in Germany, and their study in Britain did not start until 1877.

***

Developments in other fields in the 19th century facilitated the expansion of pathology. Possibly the most important early move forward was the improvements made to the compound microscope. In the late 1820s, Joseph J Lister (Lord Lister's father) solved the problem of chromatic and spherical aberration.

The first person in Britain to advocate the use of the microscope was John Hughes Bennett of Edinburgh, who, after travelling in Europe, set up the first practical classes in medical microscopy. By the time John Queckett had published his book *A practical treatise on the use of microscopes* in 1849 – the first work on specimen preparation in microtechnique – the value of microscopy in diagnosis had already been recognised.

Lionel Smith Beale set up a private laboratory near King's College Hospital in 1841, gave lectures and showed how to cut sections free hand and prepare tissue for microscopy and examine urine deposits. Later, in 1874, St Thomas' Hospital established a special course in practical microscopy related to human physiology and pathology.

However, many of the major advancements in cellular pathology were being made in Germany. Although Robert Hooke may have been the first to describe staining and van Leeuwenhoek had used saffron to stain muscle fibres, other natural dyes were used, particularly to stain plant cells, and it was the work of von Gerlach in 1858 that gave impetus to the use of dyes in histology. In the same year, Rudolf Virchow published *Die cellular pathologie*, which established cellular pathology as a vital part of a diagnostic service.

After William Perkin synthesised the first aniline dye, mauve, in 1856, many other dyes were synthesised. Although initially used on textiles, microscopists rapidly recognised the value of these dyes, and numerous staining methods were developed which allowed the clearer demonstration of the cellular anatomy of cells and their components in disease and health. Other improvements in fixation, methods for preparing sections, particularly the development of the automatic microtome, which simplified preparation of the thin even sections, and allowed ribbons of sections to be produced, gave great impetus to the development of cellular pathology.

***

It is arguable that the discovery which had the greatest impact on the need for pathology laboratories was made by Louis Pasteur. When in 1862 he showed that microorganisms were responsible for spoiling wine, he set in train a series of discoveries that led to the recognition that many diseases resulted from infection with microorganisms.

Subsequent discoveries by Robert Koch and his co-workers in Germany and researchers in the Pasteur Institute in Paris, and by many other workers in Europe, had a massive impact on the practice of medicine and public health. Joseph Lister (later Lord Lister) in Glasgow developed aseptic surgical techniques, and the understanding of how cholera and typhoid were spread led to the development of clean water and sewage systems. However, unlike most other clinical pathology investigations undertaken at the time, bacteriology could not easily be undertaken in side rooms or consulting rooms. This was well illustrated by Lister's house surgeon, William Watson

Cheyne, who, in 1876, attempted to study bacteria obtained from his chief's cases. He worked in a little passage behind the operating theatre of Edinburgh Infirmary, but without stains, oil immersion lenses, solid culture media and proper incubators.

A laboratory devoted to bacteriology research and teaching was established in 1883 by John Chiene, professor of surgery at the University of Edinburgh. However, until the late 1880s there were almost no facilities for bacteriological work in Great Britain, and anyone interested in this subject had to travel to Europe to receive training. Probably the first to study bacteriology abroad was Edgar March Crookshank, who studied with Koch in Berlin and Pasteur in Paris. On his return to England, in 1885, he published the first book on bacteriology in English. The following year he gave a lecture and demonstration on the subject to a meeting of the British Medical Association (BMA). In 1887 he started the first course in bacteriology at King's College, and courses at St Bartholomew's and Guy's hospitals followed in 1890. However, it was not until 1901 that the majority of British medical schools included bacteriology lectures in their published curricula.

***

In Scotland the establishment of a pathology laboratory was given great impetus by the visit of Louis Pasteur to Edinburgh in 1884. In the same year Professor Chiene gave a lecture to the 52nd meeting of the BMA entitled 'On the Desirability of Establishing Bacteriology Laboratories in Connection with Hospital Wards'. After protracted negotiations, The Laboratory of the Royal College of Physicians of Edinburgh was opened in 1887. Its first director was Dr German Sims Woodhead, and there were 130 applicants for the laboratory assistant posts. The purpose of the laboratory was to promote physiological and pathological investigations of specimens encountered in practice in a manner not possible or practicable in a GP's home.

In London, the Royal College of Physicians and the Royal College of Surgeons of England opened the Conjoint Laboratory in 1890, with Dr German Sims Woodhead as its director. In the same year, a bacteriology laboratory was opened in the Catholic University of Dublin. A laboratory was founded at Owens College in Manchester in 1895 by Professor Sheridan Delépine, and it pioneered the application of bacteriology to public health issues and undertook work for the Medical Officers of Health for both Manchester and Stockport. The Liverpool Pathological Diagnosis Society was established in 1887.

Following the introduction of the *Infectious Disease (Notification) Act 1889*, bacteriology services were increasingly required by Medical Officers of Health and many began to send specimens to university laboratories, but some established their own laboratories. In 1894 the Metropolitan Asylums Board in London appointed a pathologist to supervise its asylums and laboratories, and it built a modern laboratory at Claybury Hospital. In the same year, a private commercial laboratory was set up in Leicester and a pathological laboratory was established in St David's Hospital in Carmarthen, for the study of the brains of 'lunatics'. This may well be the first pathology laboratory outside a teaching hospital or royal college.

Many teaching hospitals set up clinical laboratories in the early 1890s, including Glasgow's Western Infirmary, The Brompton Hospital and St Bartholomew's, each of which had laboratories by 1893. St Thomas' Hospital and the Westminster Hospital both followed in 1897.

***

It is unclear how and why men were attracted to work in the earliest medical laboratories of this period. After all, little could have been known of the work or the conditions, and no organised training was available. Many started at an early age, often as young as 14 years, with nothing more than a limited basic education and little or no knowledge of science.

Apart from the main post of laboratory assistant, which would only be achieved after many years' experience and by an older and mature man, most entrants into medical laboratories were employed as 'lab boys'. Their role in the laboratory was to carry out any task required, many of which were menial, that might be demanded by the superintendent of the laboratory.

Lab boys received a pittance in pay, starting as low as five shillings per week. Their only chance of an increase would be if they showed particular aptitude and diligence and were noticed by the medical director of the laboratory. There was no pay structure or mechanism for pay review. It was only when a 'useful' boy looked to leave, and his absence cause inconvenience to the functioning of the laboratory, that he might be considered worthy and offered a small increase.

In spite of this situation, a small number of men developed considerable skills and a clear dedication to the work. The most famous of these early devotees was Richard Muir, whose great skill and expertise was recognised through his ultimate appointment as a demonstrator in the Edinburgh Medical School.

It is also quite clear that these workers were regarded as servants by the medical hierarchy of the laboratory, much the same as were those employed in households of the time. There is a clear reference of this in the Annual Report of the Superintendent of the RCPE Laboratory Committee for 1902, which states (with reference to laboratory assistants and boys): "Money is well spent in securing thoroughly trained servants. By doing so, busy professional men (doctors) are enabled to continue to carry out original investigations".

The post of laboratory assistant was regarded as a dead-end job, with little opportunity for progression and remuneration literally at the whim of the head of the laboratory, as was the case at the RCPE laboratory. Elsewhere, even this arrangement for pay review did not appear to exist. Laboratory workers had virtually no status or recognition in the eyes of the administrators of hospitals or universities.

There is clear evidence of the lowly status of most laboratory workers from the pay records of the time, which show that the laboratory cleaner (char lady) was paid more than the lab boys.

An enterprising laboratory man fortunate enough to find a better position would often be thwarted in his attempt to leave by his medical master, who would complain to the medical head of the recruiting institution that 'his man' was being 'poached' and the cost of his training 'wasted'. The respective heads would agree to maintain the status quo, thus denying the unfortunate assistant his chance of betterment.

This situation notwithstanding, there is evidence of genuine

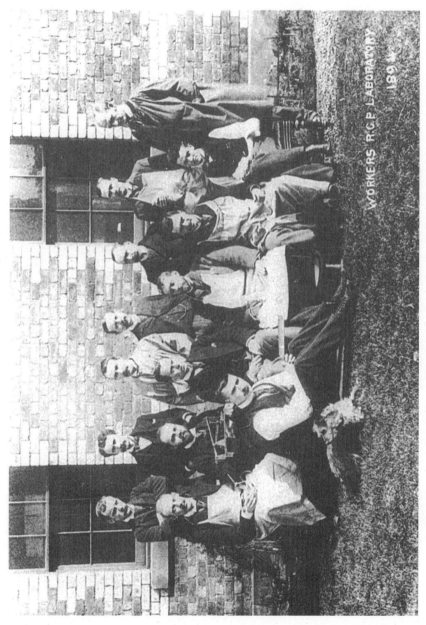

Workers in the Royal College of Physicians' laboratory in the 1890s

appreciation and allegiance demonstrated by some heads to their assistants. This was clearly apparent during the struggle to establish an association for laboratory assistants, as, in spite of fierce opposition from many senior medical figures, eminent men such as Professor Sir German Sims Woodhead and Professor James Lorrain Smith gave great support to the cause of the assistants.

***

The nature of the work undertaken during the early years in medical laboratories is worthy of note. It is clear that the original emphasis was for research, as reporting on individual samples from patients was largely performed by physicians in their own premises, with limited facilities.

The opportunity to send specimens for reporting began to put limitations on those laboratories originally established for research. The increase in specimens sent for reporting to the RCPE laboratory rose from just 50 in 1890 to over 1000 in 1898. This pattern of increase, so familiar in modern laboratories, shows how early this process began.

The range of examinations available by 1890 included urine specimens for chemical analysis, sputa for tubercle bacilli, swabs for diphtheria, blood and stool examination for typhoid, plus tumours for histological differentiation. Local authorities sought to agree arrangements for bacteriological diagnosis of infectious diseases, with the laboratory receiving a fee for each report issued.

In 1900, the Scottish authorities in Edinburgh sought agreement for cases of suspected plague to be investigated. When one considers the risks encountered by the workers – mainly laboratory assistants – carrying out these tests, the passing of the 1911 National Insurance Act was clearly overdue in providing a basic health insurance scheme for these people. There is no evidence that laboratory workers had any protection prior to this legislation.

It is interesting to see how the role of the experienced laboratory assistant had progressed since the late 1880s. In 1898, the head assistant was asked by the laboratory superintendent to go over that year's accounts and to state actual costs of, for example, materials, chemicals, coal and gas involved in carrying out the reporting work. This is probably the first example of a management exercise carried out by the laboratory staff, leading to itemised or cost-centred budgeting as it is now known.

This exercise also showed how the staff were utilised in the allocation of duties. The lab boys, the lowest paid individuals, were engaged in preparing bacteriological media, staining sputum specimens, and the assistants would be involved in the examination of the stained preparations and cultures, with those in the histopathology laboratory largely involved in section cutting. The assistants were also involved in photographic work, which, in the case of the RCPE and similar establishments, largely contributed to the research and publication of scientific papers.

***

In 1890, John McLean, of whom there will be more later, was a 'lab boy'. At just 15 years of age, but with experience, he had his pay increased to seven shillings and sixpence per week. His next rise did not come until late in the next year, when he received 10 shillings per week. Four months later he resigned his position.

Chapter 2

1911–1912

The Pathology Society of Great Britain and Ireland and the Birth of the Pathological and Bacteriological Laboratory Assistants' Association

In January 1912, a group of laboratory assistants met in Liverpool to embark on a professional voyage that had been several decades in gestation. Just over three months later, on 15 April, some 46,000 tonnes of Olympic-class vessel, the largest man-made object to have moved across the face of the earth, finally came to rest some two miles below the surface of the North Atlantic. Popularly believed to be an unsinkable vessel, the Titanic's exact resting place was not to be discovered for over 70 years.

It is perhaps fitting that the Pathological and Bacteriological Laboratory Assistants' Association (PBLAA) was both conceived and born in Liverpool. It is a city that has seen many new beginnings. As a port of embarkation, it saw many migrants leave to populate both the New World and Old World. Later it was to give the world the 'Liverpool Sound' – music that influenced and changed a generation. Neither the pop groups of Liverpool nor the 'boys' – as these mature men were often called – who formed the PBLAA had any idea that they would be so influential.

The decisions made on 6 January 1912, in the Liverpool School of Tropical Medicine, were to have far-reaching consequences. Over the last century, the Association not only developed and metamorphosed into the Institute of Biomedical Science, but also influenced and aided the formation of similar independent scientific bodies in countries that were part of the British Empire and subsequently the post-Imperial Commonwealth, and beyond.

***

Although pathology and bacteriology were becoming an increasingly important part of medical practice, even in the medical school and university laboratories there was little encouragement and less money available for teaching and research. Much of the financial burden, including the payment of assistants, often fell on the private means and income of the pathologist. Although highly valued by their laboratory 'masters', laboratory assistants were viewed as unskilled by the boards of hospitals and other controlling bodies, and, as a result, often were poorly paid when compared to other workers who enjoyed the protection of a trades union.

Opportunities for advancement were few, and even when a trained man was successful in obtaining a senior post in another laboratory, it was not uncommon for his first employer to complain to the new employer and for the contract to be withdrawn.

The situation became more difficult as increasingly high levels of knowledge, skill and reliability were required of laboratory staff, usually with no concomitant increase in status, remuneration or advancement. Thus, it became apparent that there was a need for an organisation which could represent assistants and provide employers with a method of contacting qualified and experienced men for the expanding hospital and municipal laboratory service.

***

It was against this early 20th-century pathology background that Albert Norman, who had experience in university, research, and hospital laboratories, developed the idea of forming an association of laboratory assistants. He began this daunting task by contacting as many of his colleagues as possible – no mean feat when one considers the limited means of communication available – seeking their views on the formation of an association of assistants working in pathology and bacteriology. Norman recognised that a militant approach would be counterproductive, and for the organisation to be a success it needed to benefit both employer and employee.

Although he was clear that any association formed must be organised for and by the assistants themselves, it was essential that it had the goodwill of those in high places. To ensure this, he discussed his ideas with the eminent pathologists with whom he had come in contact, and also took advice from members of the then newly formed Pathological Society of Great Britain and Ireland (PathSoc). He was quite clear that the cooperation and support of the Society would be essential and therefore sought its assistance in forming an association of assistants in pathology and bacteriology. At the same time he requested recognition of its status and aims, thereby preventing any misconception as to the nature of the movement, which otherwise might have been thought to be of a militant trades union character.

It was Albert Norman's previous boss, Professor James Lorrain Smith, who undertook to bring the project to the attention of the PathSoc committee. Professor Lorrain Smith, who was to become the new association's first President, had played a prominent role in formation of the PathSoc in 1906. Unsurprisingly, many of its members viewed the proposal with distrust, but the majority of members soon realised that the association could perform a useful role, especially helping to solve the pressing problems

A PROPOSAL TO FORM AN ASSOCIATION OF ASSISTANTS IN PATHOLOGICAL & BACTERIOLOGICAL LABORATORIES AND MUSEUMS

DEAR SIR,

We beg to ask your consideration of the proposal to form an Association of Assistants in Pathological and Bacteriological Laboratories and Museums.

Some of the objects of the Association would be (i) to form a means of communication amongst the assistants in these laboratories, (ii) to supply to the members information regarding appointments, and (iii) to assist members by circulating information regarding the most recent methods, modifications of methods, and matter of general interest.

At present there is no recognized means of dealing with any of these objects, and the difficulties connected with them would, it is hoped, be in a large measure solved by means of the proposed Association.

It is further suggested that the Association should work in conjunction with the Pathological Society of Great Britain and Ireland, the Council of which has appointed a sub-committee to assist in its formation.

A large number of assistants have already agreed to the proposal, but before giving the matter more definite shape we are endeavouring to ascertain the views of assistants in all the Pathological and Bacteriological laboratories and museums in the country.

We should be glad to hear that you are willing to join the Association as an Original Member, and should welcome any suggestion you may have to make as to the Constitution of the Association.

A provisional committee will be elected to draft the Constitution of the Association, and in the event of your deciding to become a member, we should be glad if you will suggest six names for this committee.

It might be pointed out that, although at first it is proposed to confine the membership to assistants in Pathology and Bacteriology, it is hoped eventually to have an Association which shall include all laboratory assistants.

As we are anxious to hold the first Committee meeting at Liverpool on January 6th, 1912 when the Pathological Society meets there you will greatly oblige by replying to this circular at your earliest convenience, so that necessary arrangements may be made.

We are.

Yours faithfully,

F. G. HALLIDAY, Liverpool; F. A. IZZARD, Cambridge; WM. MANEY, Manchester; W. A. MITCHELL, Cambridge; J. MOSS, London; R. MUIR, Edinburgh; A. NORMAN, Liverpool: R. N. STEVEN, Belfast; R. B. SUTTON, London; W. WATSON, Edinburgh; E. WHEAL, Oxford.

If it is your intention to join the Association, kindly fill in and forward the enclosed post-card

---

The letter circulated by Albert Norman and others in 1911.

of training and remuneration, the solution to which would eventually lead to an end to the 'blind alley' problem.

At a meeting of its committee, held in Oxford in July 1911, the PathSoc appointed a subcommittee consisting of Professor Lorrain Smith, Dr Boycott and Dr Ledingham "to consider the formation of an employment bureau for laboratory assistants". Following these discussions, a circular letter was sent to all the laboratory workers who could be traced.

***

There are no records showing how many pathology laboratories were operating in the British Isles in 1911 when Albert Norman revived John McLean's idea of an association for laboratory assistants working in pathology and bacteriology laboratories. In 1910/1911, the PathSoc had about 250 members. As this was the only learned society devoted exclusively to the study of pathology at this time, it is reasonable to assume that this number represented most of the pathology laboratories in the British Isles. These laboratories were mainly, but not exclusively, situated in universities and medical schools. In the register of members of the PathSoc not all members gave their laboratory as their address, but using those who did, plus tracing others through their publications and adding those laboratories that were known to exist, it is possible to identify 65 individual laboratories. Some of these may have been physiology and pharmacology departments, and can be excluded, but other unidentified departments may have existed.

So, in 1911, there were probably between 60 and 70 laboratories that employed laboratory assistants eligible for membership of the proposed association when Albert Norman and the others sent out their circular. The response they received was encouraging. A total of 170 letters were distributed and 120 assistants replied expressing an interest. This would have represented a significant proportion of those working in the field at the time.

The letter brought the plans to the attention of John McLean, who, in 1896, had attempted to form an organisation for all assistants in medical laboratories, the role of which was to act as both an employment register and a means of communication for the assistants. Sadly, McLean's original letter to Professor German Sims Woodhead is lost in the mists of time, but Sims Woodhead's reply demonstrates sympathy with McLean's ideas. Unfortunately, the attempt was unsuccessful. Nevertheless, McLean gave wholehearted support to Albert Norman's efforts in forming an association.

Not all those contacted supported the formation of an association. Some well-established men believed that it was not needed and would not benefit them. Others did not believe their 'chiefs' would allow them to join, but others wanted to join because their 'chiefs' told them not to join, while some would not join as they felt it was bound to fail. With the notable exceptions of John McLean and Richard Muir, many older men did not join, and many younger men followed their lead. The men who laid the foundations of the association were nearly all in their thirties. Surprisingly, a significant number of responses to the letter came from workers in Sydney, Australia, and subsequently a thriving branch of the new association was established in New South Wales.

***

A provisional committee of the new Pathological and Bacteriological Laboratory Assistants' Association (PBLAA) was formed following a postcard ballot of those wishing to join the embryonic association. Those elected were R Muir (Edinburgh), R B Sutton (London), F A Izzard (Cambridge), W A Mitchell (Cambridge), E Wheal (Oxford), W Manby (Manchester) and A Norman (Liverpool). Its first meeting was held on Saturday 6 January 1912 in Liverpool, following a PathSoc meeting. Earlier that day, the provisional committee had informal discussions with a PathSoc subcommittee.

The members of the provisional committee present at the first meeting were Messrs. Izzard, Manby, Muir and Norman. Richard Muir was elected Chairman, and Albert Norman Honorary Secretary and Treasurer. Five other members attended this first meeting: P Duncan (Liverpool), G F Garner (Birmingham), R Frost (Sheffield), D Peden (Liverpool) and J McLean (London). John McLean was coopted as an addition committee member for the London District.

In addition to the appointment of the committee, a general outline of the objects and constitution of the PBLAA was drawn up and discussed. However, agreement on the final wording took several months. It should be remembered that all of this was achieved when telephones were still uncommon – making calls from city to city was by prebooked trunk call, and email and internet facilities were still many decades in the future. The only method of communication open to the members of the PBLAA committee was by letter as round-the-table discussions were not possible.

However, after considerable deliberation and consultation with other assistants, the results of their efforts, together with an account of the inaugural meeting, were reported in July 1912 in *The Journal of the Pathological and Bacteriology Assistants' Association*. As the Provisional Committee agreed that the objectives of the PBLAA would be best served through the medium of a 'Monthly Journal', it was decided to issue the report in the Journal. The rules drawn up are shown in the Appendix, but perhaps the most important and enduring of these are the objectives of the Association set out in Rule 2, as follows:

- To form a means of communication amongst the assistants
- To supply information regarding appointments
- To assist in the general advancement of its members.

The wording was clear in intent but sufficiently open to allow intelligent interpretation. Arguably, these broad principles became, and remain, the rationale for all the activities of the PBLAA and of its successor bodies over the past century.

Professor Lorrain Smith and John McLean set out their views as to the value of the newly formed PBLAA. Although looking at its formation from different professional standpoints, their views were similar. Both emphasised that it was essential that laboratory assistants be recognised as skilled and knowledgeable men, and that the PBLAA could play a role in this respect. They agreed that there was a need for a system to facilitate the advertising of vacancies – a benefit both to employers and to those seeking promotion.

They also believed that the PBLAA would be an important conduit for the exchange of ideas and information between assistants, and provide a mechanism for building unity within the nascent profession. To further these aims it was decided that a 'Monthly Journal' should be produced. This would not only provide a mechanism for informing members of developments within the PBLAA but also provide a vehicle for advertising vacancies as well as a means to publish articles on technical and scientific developments and practices.

It was further agreed that the PBLAA should comprise four Divisions and that each should appoint members to represent them on the Association's committee. These were Division A (London and District), Division B (Cambridge, Bristol, Cardiff and Norwich), Division C (Manchester, Liverpool, Sheffield, Leeds and Newcastle on Tyne), and Division D (Scotland and Ireland). London and District was to have two representatives, and the other Divisions one each. These decisions laid the foundations that, although modified over the years, still form the basis for the exchange of information.

***

Although soundly established, the PBLAA was not without its problems, and the report concluded with an appeal for members to pay their subscriptions and by so doing help to pay the expenses so far incurred, mainly out of the pockets of the founders. On a more positive note, there was a report that Arthur Haywood of the Westminster Hospital had been appointed, through the agency of the PBLAA, to the post of senior laboratory assistant in the University of Bristol. Equally encouraging was the first advertisement of a vacancy for a fully trained assistant to work in the Cancer Research Laboratory in the Pathological Department of the University of Manchester – this post was filled by a PBLAA member. Sadly, Mr Haywood, the successful candidate for the vacancy in Bristol, was not a PBLAA member and, although he promised to do so, he never joined the Association.

Chapter 3

Founding Fathers

McLean, Sims Woodhead, Lorrain Smith, Muir and Norman, too

The years straddling the turn of the 20th century are referred to as the Edwardian era, but also known as La Belle Epoque. The British Empire was at the peak of its power. Edward VII replaced Victoria in 1901, but his long-awaited reign was all too short. Victoria's descendents in the royal houses of Europe were dominant influences on events during the first decade of the century. Nonetheless, the wind of change was picking up, as events and personalities in pathology were soon to demonstrate.

John McLean (1875–1963) was the first medical laboratory worker to propose the benefits of forming an Association for his fellow laboratory assistants.

John was born in Edinburgh and started work at the age of 14 after only basic schooling. He was recruited as a 'lab boy' at five shillings (25 pence) per week in the laboratory of the Royal College of Physicians of Edinburgh (RCPE) in 1889.

Records of the laboratory committee of the RCPE show that such was his aptitude and progress that in May 1890, aged 15, he was recognised as the 'elder laboratory boy' – in other words, experienced – and had his pay increased by 50%. He received a further increase in 1892, and this should be seen in the context of the fact that there were no pay scales or automatic increases at this time. Lab boys would be paid as little as possible and would only receive an increase at the behest of the laboratory director. Despite this modest recognition, McLean, seeing no opportunity to gain a post as a full assistant, decided to move to Birmingham as an assistant to Professor Leith at University College.

During his early years at RCPE, McLean worked under the direction of Dr German Sims Woodhead, who later became director of laboratories of the Conjoint Board of the Royal College of Surgeons and Physicians in London. In 1896, John McLean wrote to Dr Sims Woodhead to seek his backing to form an association of laboratory assistants in pathology laboratories. Regrettably, his original letter is lost, but the well-considered and clear aim of his intentions, described in his later correspondence, delivered at the formation of the Pathological and Bacteriological Laboratory Assistants' Association (PBLAA), are clear to see.

The Association considered from the Assistants' point of view

The formation of a laboratory assistants' association has long been a desirable object, and of late years has become more and more a necessity. It is sometimes asked – "What would be the advantage of such an Association?" and although these ought to be obvious, I might just briefly state some of them from the assistants' point of view.

First of all, it is desirable that the laboratory assistant should be recognised as a skilled worker. Professors, lecturers and other scientists connected with the various subjects included in the medical curriculum do recognise this fact, but there are others, some of whom are members of the committee of management of our various universities, hospitals and research laboratories, who seem to be under the impression that no skill or special knowledge is required of the laboratory assistant, and that his work is more or less unskilled and purely mechanical.

Our association will endeavour to convince them of their mistake and will, further, work to improve the status of the laboratory assistant. I do not mean to infer that our movement is one of militant trade unionism; that is neither necessary nor expedient.

Our association will also provide a means of registration and a medium whereby a member may get into communication with others on matters of interest. At present, the laboratory assistant is much handicapped in his search for an opportunity to better himself by this lack of registration, and he has no recognised medium whereby he may obtain the desired information. The employer seeking a skilled and specially trained assistant has a similar difficulty to contend with, so that it often happens that 'out of works' of various callings with no previous laboratory training are taken on simply because of this lack of registration, and a common centre through which the employer may get in touch with the man he requires. The laboratory boy spends the most critical years of his life training to become a skilled laboratory assistant, and I would ask – "Is it right, that some unemployed white-washer should stand as much chance of laboratory employment as the fully trained youth?" These are real grievances which have required redressing for many years, and they cannot be allowed to go on longer.

Then there is the social side of the movement. Many of us have to do much routine work and are inclined to get into a groove; we require to mix more with our fellow workers so that we may compare details of methods, learning from the experience of others where our own technique may be improved; and at the same time have the opportunity of helping those who may have difficulties. Opportunities of forming new friendships will be obtained, all the more likely to be lasting because of our common interests. Most of us, I hope, are not so much in need of help and sympathy, but happily, may be in a position to extend the same.

If the question arises: "Is the Association going to benefit me?" and the answer seems doubtful, ask also: "Is it going to benefit the younger members?" There can be no doubt of that answer and there should be no hesitation in deciding to become a member of the association. Rest assured that time will show how helpful such an association will prove to all its members.

Dr Sims Woodhead was most supportive of McLean's original proposal, as can be seen by his reply, sent on 24 November 1896.

My Dear McLean,

There can be no doubt that such an association as you mention, if worked on proper lines, would be of immense advantage to those engaged in laboratory work. By a system of registration, local and central, it would be possible to keep thoroughly in touch with one another, whilst now that the laboratories are becoming more numerous and better developed, the special training of assistants is a subject that will come prominently forward, and, as much of the training has to be done by the senior laboratory assistants, an association with definite objectives and rules would be able to ensure regular and systemic instruction for those who intended to keep to the work, whilst the system of registration would ensure the claims of men who had been specially trained would always receive due consideration. It would be well, however, that you should remember that such banding together, if it is to be of any use, must be entirely voluntary and absolutely free from compulsion; that absence of voluntarism is the rock on which all these things split. If any association were well managed on such lines, I believe it would be of great advantage to laboratory assistants and also to those by whom they are employed.

With kindest regards

I am

Yours faithfully

G Sims Woodhead

London

Despite his position and reputation, Sims Woodhead could not engender a majority of medical support for McLean's plan at this time (1896). It took a further 16 years for the eventual founding of the Pathological and Bacteriological Laboratory Assistants' Association by Albert Norman, with continued support from German Sims Woodhead.

Although John McLean was not among the original signatories to the formation of the PBLAA in 1912, he was very enthusiastic towards the new organisation and was immediately co-opted to the Provisional Committee as an additional member for the London District, where at that time he was working and living. He was the first chairman of the London branch and a member of the Executive Council from 1915 and again in 1921–1938, and succeeded Richard Muir as PBLAA Vice President in 1916, serving in this role until 1920. McLean and Muir were the first Life Members of the PBLAA.

McLean was a member of the Examining Council from 1921 until the formation of the Institute of Medical Laboratory Technology (IMLT) in 1942, when he was persuaded to carry on as a member of the Examining Body (Final) to assist during the difficult wartime years.

Following the incorporation of the IMLT, McLean was elected a Vice President of the new body in 1942. He retired from Institute activities in 1948 but continued to take a keen interest in developments up to the time of his death in 1963.

***

German Sims Woodhead (1855–1921) was professor of pathology in the University of Cambridge from 1899 and PBLAA president in 1916–1922. Professor Sir German Sims Woodhead was very influential in the formation of the PBLAA. His support to Richard Muir and Albert Norman, and his eminent position within the Pathological Society of Great Britain and Ireland, helped to make possible the eventual establishment of the Association.

German Sims Woodhead was born near Huddersfield in Yorkshire, the son of a Member of Parliament, who later became editor and proprietor of the *Huddersfield Examiner* newspaper. He was educated in Huddersfield before going to the University of Edinburgh, where he qualified in medicine in 1878. Devoted to his studies, Sims Woodhead attained his MD four years later and was elected a Fellow of Royal College of Physicians of Edinburgh (RCPE) in 1882 after studying in Berlin and Vienna.

Sims Woodhead was appointed the first superintendent of the RCPE laboratories in 1887 and remained there until 1890. During his tenure he encountered an able 'laboratory boy' named John McLean and also Richard Muir who was well established at this time, working at the medical school in Edinburgh.

Sims Woodhead was a founder member of the PathSoc in 1906 and gave continuing support to laboratory staff when, in 1911–12, new attempts to form an Association took place. He was, perhaps, one of the central pillars of medical support, with Lorrain Smith, in overcoming the prejudice and opposition which obstructed earlier efforts. This eventually resulted in the PathSoc laying a path for discussions and subsequent formation of the PBLAA by Richard Muir, Albert Norman and colleagues.

Sims Woodhead, always a keen volunteer for military activity, offered his services at the outbreak of war in 1914. He held several positions in the War Office and his work on chlorination of water supplies was of benefit at home and overseas. In 1919 he received a knighthood, being appointed KBE (Knight Commander of the British Empire) for his extensive military services. He had a long association with the diagnosis and treatment of tuberculosis, which he continued throughout his life, publishing many papers and leading many studies, including a Royal Commission.

Professor Sir German Sims Woodhead will forever feature as a key figure in the history of the Institute, from the formation of its predecessor, the PBLAA, right through to the present day, when the commemorative award and medal, established in his name, remains the highest accolade accorded by the Institute.

***

James Lorrain Smith (1862–1931) was professor of pathology and Dean of the Faculty of Medicine in the University of Edinburgh, and the first president of the Pathological and Bacteriological Laboratory Assistants' Association.

James Lorrain Smith was born near Dumfries in Scotland, in 1862, the fourth son of a Free Church minister. He went on to achieve outstanding academic and medical qualifications at Edinburgh, Oxford and Cambridge universities, firstly in philosophy in 1884 before embarking on his first medical studies, graduating with first-class honours in 1888. He proceeded to the University of Oxford, working and teaching under the tutelage of Professor Burdon-Sanderson and later with Dr J S Haldane, collaborating in a series of physiological studies on respiratory function and the oxygen capacity of blood.

In 1893, Lorrain Smith moved to Cambridge, gaining an MD a year later.

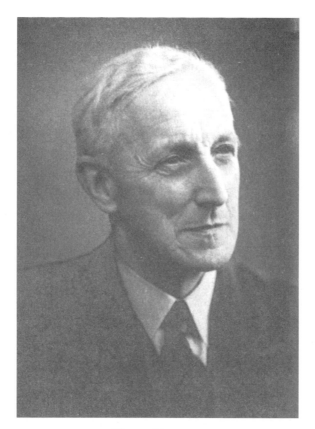

Albert Norman

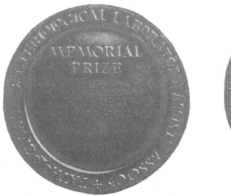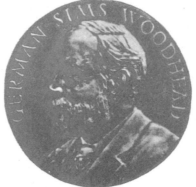

Sims Woodhead Medal

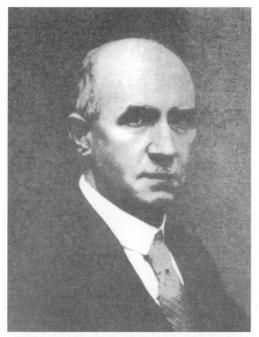

John McLean

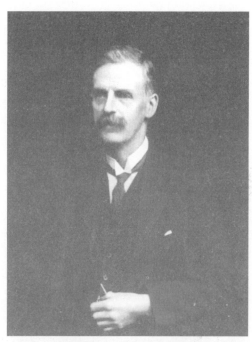

James Lorrain Smith

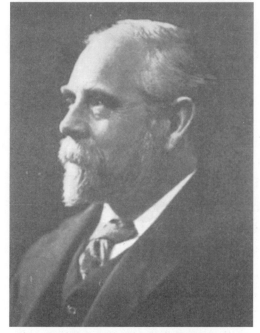

German Sims Woodhead

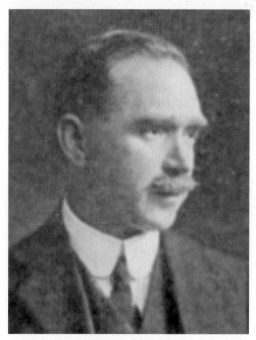

Richard Muir

During his period at Cambridge, the direction of his career moved fully to the study of pathology. He gained his first appointment in pathology at Queen's College, Belfast, in 1895, and such was his progress that he attained the status of professor during his tenure there.

Professor Lorrain Smith was appointed to the chair of pathology at the University of Manchester in 1904. It was during this appointment, which is of most significance to the formation of the PBLAA, that Albert Norman became steward of Lorrain Smith's laboratory in 1907. Norman became Lorrain Smith's personal assistant for the next four years until the former moved to Liverpool in 1911.

There can be little doubt that their relationship paved the way towards achieving the support in medical circles for the founding of the PBLAA. It was Lorrain Smith who, as an esteemed and highly respected founder member of the PathSoc, undertook to bring the proposals for the new Association (PBLAA) to the notice of the Society's Committee in July 1911. This was the most important act in gaining the vital backing needed to float the embryonic assistants' association. Following the formation of the PBLAA at the meeting of the PathSoc in Liverpool in January 1912, Professor Lorrain Smith agreed to become its first president, serving in this role until 1915.

Lorrain Smith's many scientific contributions included the series of studies on the physiology and pathology of respiratory function, the oxygen capacity of blood (with J S Haldane) and the determination of blood volume. He was remembered by many laboratory workers for his study of the metabolism of fat and its pathological identification in tissues. In 1908 he described the Nile blue staining method, used to distinguish fatty acids and neutral fats, which was used regularly for this purpose for many years.

During the First World War he was invited to investigate sepsis in wounds and seek a practical form of antiseptic for military use. This resulted in his identification of the use of hypochlorite and the introduction of Evsol, which became widely used as an antiseptic agent.

Lorrain Smith was a thoughtful and considerate man, taken to thoughtful reflection rather than outspoken comment, but he proved to be an outstanding leader in medicine, especially in the field of education. His affection with laboratory life and its members led him to give his great support to the formation of the PBLAA and ultimately the Institute.

***

Richard Muir (1862–1931) was demonstrator of pathological and bacteriological methods at the University of Edinburgh Medical School. He was the elder statesman of the fledgling association of laboratory assistants, which became the PBLAA. He was originally employed as 'lab boy' but, through his skills and dedication, became a revered figure in the University of Edinburgh Medical School.

Richard Muir was born in Edinburgh in 1862 and remained in his native city throughout his career and his life. He was one of the first 'lab boys', appointed in Edinburgh in 1877 by Dr D J Hamilton, assistant to Professor Sanders in the University Medical School. His engagement was coincidental with the establishment of the first practical classes in pathology in Great Britain.

Muir's skills were recognised by Dr Hamilton and, through his contributions to teaching and research in pathology at Edinburgh University Medical School, he was appointed as a University Demonstrator by the University Court. Further recognition followed when he was elected a member of the PathSoc in 1908, believed to be the first non-medically qualified member.

Richard Muir was one of the original signatories to the proposal to form the PBLAA and was invited to join the working party with the PathSoc to further the project. He is recorded as the first member of the PBLAA (Member No 001) and became its first Vice President.

It is believed that Muir agreed personally to underwrite the financial stability of the PBLAA during the early days when there was little or no income before any subscriptions were received. Such was his generosity and dedication to his colleagues.

Among his many skills, Muir was an accurate scientific artist in his depiction of microscopy images. In 1911 he was invited to compile a section on pathology in the 5th edition of *Encyclopaedia Britannica*. In 1927 he published *Muir's Bacteriological Atlas*, presenting his fine drawings of bacteria and other microscopy images of cells and organisms, which he had produced earlier as part of his teaching materials.

There is no doubt that Muir was held in great esteem by the many medical students who passed through his careful tuition, which is described in an article published in the students' university magazine, *Gambolier*, in 1910.

Richard Muir

As one, in early student days, passes up to the pathological department, one occasionally catches a glimpse of an inner door which bears the inscription 'Richard Muir'. The words for a time cause a passing wonder for an element of mystery centres around the name associated in the students mind with numerous staining methods; only when one begins to battle with practical work have they a vivid meaning, for then they are embodied in a silently moving, unobtrusive figure, whose characteristic question "Are you in any difficulty?" and "What can I do to assist you?" are at once followed by equally characteristic deeds. To the old student, too, the chief memory recalled by the mention of his name is of ever-willing and ever-skillful pilot. It is after one comes into closer touch with Richard Muir, however, that there is laid fully bare not merely the extraordinary skill of the man, but also his courtesy, his delicacy of feeling, his generosity of thought and act. Class assistants and research workers are proud to owe their dependence on him for scientific light and leading always modestly bestowed. Former class assistants, now famous, such as Sims Woodhead, Alexis Thompson and Beattie, honour him as a friend and consult him as an oracle. And to many able workers throughout the world, who have never seen his face, his name is a laboratory word.

'University Demonstrator of Pathological and Bacteriological Methods' is the academic title of Richard Muir, but the words in no way adequately suggest his varied work as postgraduate lecturer, examiner of pathological material, photographer of microscopy subjects, illustrator of books and theses which are lit up by his genius, chooser and preparer of specimens – probably the finest in the world – for the classes and demonstrations and general advisor to workers far and near. Neither would his title in itself lead anyone to expect that its holder is the writer of the article on pathology in the forthcoming edition of the *Encyclopaedia Britannica*.

The work of Richard Muir is unique and so is his life story. As a boy of thirteen, with ordinary education incomplete, and with no scientific education, he entered the pathological laboratory. To the wise enthusiasm and scientific genius of Dr Hamilton, at that time assistant to Professor Saunders, he owes the foundation of what he is as a scientist and artist, and to his present revered chief who developed Hamilton's work he acknowledges an even greater debt. A man of no hobbies, except photography, Richard Muir is above all things a lover of his work and a lover of his fellow man. And those who know him know that the scientific spirit has not destroyed but only deepened the natural humility of a devout spirit that makes him also a lover of God. For him, if of anyone, it may be said "Never work like his was done for work's ignoble sake: men need a finer aim to light and lure".

Richard Muir shared an intriguing fact of his life with another, in that he was born and died in the same years as his eminent colleague and head of faculty, Professor James Lorrain Smith.

***

Albert Norman MBE (1882–1964) is widely regarded as the founder of the PBLAA in 1912, which became incorporated as the Institute of Medical Laboratory Technology (IMLT) in 1942. He held every position of office open to him in both the PBLAA and the IMLT.

Albert Norman was born in 1882 near Cambridge, the son of a farm worker. At the age of 14 he began working in the Zoological Laboratory of Cambridge University as a 'lab boy'. He learned histological techniques and gained experience in taxidermy. After three years he transferred to the university pathology department where he learned bacteriological and pathological methods. It is at this time that he probably made his first influential contact with Professor Sims Woodhead, who had just been appointed to the chair in pathology at Cambridge in 1899.

He spent just three months at Cambridge before moving to the Norfolk and Norwich Hospital, where he was the sole laboratory worker, assisting physicians and surgeons in developing the laboratory for diagnostic work. Norman enjoyed over five years at Norwich, continuing to expand his knowledge and experience. He undertook museum preparation, radiography and even assisted in the hospital pharmacy.

In 1905 Norman moved on to Edinburgh, where he stayed for two years before gaining a significant appointment to the pathology department of Victoria University in Manchester. In Manchester, Norman was to encounter a second major influence in Professor Lorrain Smith – the professor of pathology and his head of department who would become his greatest ally in his quest to organise an association for laboratory assistants.

Albert Norman was very aware of the low regard given to his colleagues, being considered as unskilled; their prospects were bleak with poor remuneration. This unjust situation motivated him to seek formal training and qualifications towards gaining professional status, as the scope of skills demanded of laboratory workers was, in contrast, constantly rising.

Lorrain Smith was, as an influential founder member of the Pathological Society of Great Britain and Ireland, pivotal in engendering the support of PathSoc members to agree to hold exploratory meetings with Albert Norman and Richard Muir, from which the PBLAA was conceived. It was Norman's relationship with such key people that enabled the embryonic PBLAA to go forward in the most difficult years of the First World War.

Norman's penultimate career move was from Manchester to Liverpool, where he was working at the time of the formation of the PBLAA. He became the chief assistant at the pathological laboratory of the Department of Obstetrics and Gynaecology at the University of Liverpool. It is of note that his new chief, Professor Harry Briggs, was a student under the guidance of Lord Lister while studying in Edinburgh.

In 1913 Albert Norman made his final move to the post that he was to hold for almost 40 years. He was appointed chief laboratory assistant at the Board of Agriculture and Fisheries at Weybridge, Surrey. His knowledge resulted in him becoming very influential in developing and planning new veterinary laboratories throughout the United Kingdom.

Norman served on the government-commissioned Cope Committee, investigating the training and recruitment of medical laboratory technicians. He was also a member of the working party invited to contribute to the Draft Bill which became the *Professions Supplementary to Medicine Act 1960*. Norman also carried out two assignments in Europe for the Food and

Agricultural Organisation, a United Nations appointment in the early 1960s.

In 1962, the Institute held a celebratory dinner at the Golden Jubilee Triennial Conference in Edinburgh. In his presidential address, Professor H A Magnus said: "Your profession owes its greatest debt of all to Mr Albert Norman MBE, whom we are delighted to see here today. All his adult life, Albert Norman has devoted his time, his energy and great diplomatic skill and charm in the furtherance of the status of the medical laboratory technician."

Albert Norman attended his last meeting of the IMLT Council's General Purposes Committee only shortly before his death in his 83rd year, and died on 22 December 1964 on the Isle of Wight.

In 1982, a Centenary Dinner was held at Trinity College, Cambridge, on 16 July, to commemorate the birth, near Cambridge, of Albert Norman on 18 July 1882.

Chapter 4

1912–1924
Of War and Women

The low country of northern France and southern Belgium is redolent of a period of history anchored in monochrome images of carnage on an almost unimaginable scale. The First World War cast a blight across the early years of the reign of King George V and was responsible for significant change, both in society and politics. During the four years of conflict, a generation of young men was decimated, and the role of women began to change.

As a result of much hard work during the previous year, the first annual meeting of the PBLAA committee was held on Saturday 4 January 1913. Albert Norman presented a lengthy written report on the activities of the Provisional Committee and the financial statement for 1912. Although not all of those who initially expressed an interest in joining eventually did so, by the end of 1912 there were 117 members, including 21 Juniors. At this meeting it was agreed to accept members from outside the UK and, where possible, invite them to form branches. Three overseas applicants were accepted – one each from Canada, Ceylon and Sudan.

It was unanimously agreed to invite Professor James Lorrain Smith to become the first PBLAA President. In extending the invitation, the committee expressed its gratitude for his help in the formation of the Association. Richard Muir was invited to become Vice President, as were a number of prominent pathologists. They also agreed that, during their term of office, the Honorary Secretaries and Honorary Treasurer of the PathSoc should be made Honorary Members, thus helping to cement a formal link between the two bodies that was to last for many years.

The rules, with some minor amendments, were approved. As it was discovered that non-members had successfully applied for vacancies advertised through the Association, it was agreed that advertisements of vacancies should show only the District, qualifications and the approximate salary for the post. Members who were interested in the post could then obtain full information about it from the Divisional or the Honorary Secretary.

A total of 32 vacancies were advertised in 1914 and Albert Norman reported that he had been instrumental, in several instances, in obtaining an increase in the salary offered. He also took the view that employers who advertised through the PBLAA did so in the belief that it could supply the genuine article and that being a member of the Association was a guarantee of competence.

***

At the beginning of 1914 the membership had reached 136, including members in Australia, Canada, Sudan and New Zealand. However, the hard work and enthusiasm of the founders notwithstanding, the Association could not be described as healthy. It had run for two years on one year's subscriptions and these were insufficient to cover the cost of the organisation and printing the *The Laboratory Journal*. Fortunately, the income from advertisements was sufficient to cover the deficit.

The situation was made worse by the outbreak of war, and, as members either volunteered or were conscripted into the forces, the income from subscriptions fell. As the war progressed it was realised that at the end of the conflict there would probably be a large number of 'war-trained' men returning to laboratories. The officers of the PBLAA felt it was their duty to ensure that the organisation remained financially sound. Subscription income fell from £32 in 1914 to £5 15s (£5 75p) in 1918, as, in common with other bodies, members were excused from paying subscriptions while on war service.

Fortunately, as the result of Albert Norman's hard work in canvassing for advertisements for the *The Laboratory Journal*, the organisation remained not only solvent but was able to show a surplus of £78 15s 7½p (£78.78p) in 1919. It was the committee's intention to use this money to help fund the introduction of a certification scheme, the details of which started to be developed in 1916. In spite of the difficulties, the editor managed to keep publishing *The Laboratory Journal* until 1917, but, due to the high cost of printing and the need to conserve money for the certification scheme, publication was suspended until 1921.

***

In 1916 Professor Sir German Sims Woodhead became President and remained in the position until his untimely death in December 1920. It is to the credit of the committee and the Officers of the Association that they managed to keep things going during the war period, even managing to hold annual meetings in 1915 and 1916; however, no further meetings were held until November 1920.

The 1920 annual meeting was an important one for the future development of the Association and the profession. It appointed the

Certification Subcommittee; established, in conjunction with the PathSoc, the first Examining Council; created the grades of Life Member and Associate Member; and agreed that general meetings of Members of the Association should be held annually in convenient centres on invitation from local branches.

***

At the start of the First World War in 1914, the committee recognised that in previous conflicts disease caused many deaths to both combatants and civilians. It therefore suggested that members should not enlist but keep their skills available until it was clear how they could be used to best advantage. However, this was thought by many to be unpatriotic and by December 1914 at least 32 members were reported to be "on service", and one member, Mr J Connor of the Highland Light Infantry, had been wounded. By 1917 it was known that at least 83 members had joined up and by end of the conflict the membership records show that at least six members had been killed. What proportion of the membership this represented is unclear.

What is apparent is that a high proportion of those who joined up were attached to fighting regiments rather than to the Royal Army Medical Corps (RAMC). While for some this may have been a matter of choice, for most it may well have resulted from the Army's unwillingness to recognise their training and skills.

At the outbreak of the war, PBLAA membership included a significant proportion of the civilian skilled pathological and bacteriological assistants in the country. The Association approached the medical authorities at the War Office offering the services of trained assistants to help train military laboratory assistants. Unfortunately, the authorities took the view that these men had no special skills and often ignored the correspondence. Indeed, the Honorary Secretary was told to his face by a senior army officer that his members were merely unskilled menials.

Undaunted, further contacts were made through the good offices of the PBLAA President, who approached various bodies including the Director General of Recruiting, but these approaches were also rebuffed. When an approach was made to General Sir Alfred Keogh, Surgeon General and Director of the RAMC, he replied that the RAMC was closed for recruiting!

It was not the PBLAA's intention to prevent members joining the armed forces, rather its aim was to ensure that highly trained men were used to the best possible advantage. However, for whatever reason, the Army chose not to use them as fully as they might have done. On occasions, rather peculiar decisions were made, such as the case of a tailor appointed to a military laboratory because he had taken up microscopy as a hobby.

For many years the relationship between the PBLAA and the British Army was somewhat strained. The problems started in 1913 when a number of applications were received from naval and military laboratory attendants. However, these men were not eligible for membership as they had not had three years training – the training period for servicemen at that time was as little as six and no more than eighteen months – and the Association was a civilian organisation. When men from the forces were told this, several attempted to bring pressure on the PBLAA by stating that they had been recommended and supported by 'prominent pathologists'.

Members working in Cambridge went so far as to write to Sims Woodhead about their concerns, which centred on their understanding that the army men's sole purpose for joining was to use the Association purely as an employment exchange. In the view of the Cambridge members, there were already sufficient bodies to look after the welfare of ex-servicemen, and that these men often obtained advancement for 'patriotic motives'.

They also pointed out that a major purpose of the Association was educational, not just to provide an employment exchange. They were concerned that should the Association be pressured into accepting Army personnel on equal terms to those who had civilian training that this would "menace seriously the future of laboratory youth" who were already in what had been described as 'blind alley' employment.

This letter, and the problem it described, was discussed at the annual meeting of the committee in January 1914 and a proposal from Mr Mitchell – "That it is considered advisable in the interests of the Association, and especially of the younger members thereof, that in future the period of training to qualify for ordinary membership be raised from three years to five years and Rule 3a be amended to that effect" – was passed unanimously. This alteration did not affect the then current Junior Members who would still become Ordinary Members when they reached 20 years of age.

These differences were resolved in 1922 when Sergeant Major Steele wrote to the Association requesting that members of the RAMC be admitted as members. Following further correspondence and discussion, it was agreed that those military personnel in possession of the RAMC certificate who had three years' laboratory experience from the date of the RAMC certificate would be admitted as Ordinary Members.

***

It would seem that the War Office was more sympathetic to the profession and to pathology some two decades later in 1938. Several members wrote to the Association asking whether the authorities had been approached regarding the duties of laboratory technicians if war broke out. The Honorary Secretary at that time, Sidney J Denyer, wrote to the War Office to inform it that there were 1200 trained and trainee laboratory technicians in the Association. After briefly explaining the training and PBLAA certification system and the problems encountered during the First World War, he suggested that emergency requirements for laboratory technicians could be met by the Association. A reply was received within two weeks, which indicated that consideration was being given to the best use of the members if war broke out. Indeed, at about this time, Dr Panton and Dr Topley were compiling a record of all UK pathologists and medical laboratory technicians in preparation for the outbreak of hostilities.

***

Throughout this period, members of the Association and laboratory assistants generally were referred to as men or boys, simply because until the beginning of the 1920s the PBLAA had no lady members. At a meeting of Division D held in Edinburgh on 28 May 1921 a motion to admit ladies as members of the Association was proposed by Mr Watson and seconded by Mr Barr. This was accepted. Subsequently, at a meeting of the PBLAA committee on 4 February

1922 in London, it was reported that a proposal to admit women to membership of the Association had been considered by the Divisions and was carried by 48 votes to 26, but in reality the majority was much greater as two of the Divisions had passed the motion unanimously. Not all members were in favour of admitting women to the Association, as they would take men's jobs.

This discussion implies that there must have been a number of women working in the laboratories of these Divisions and that the quality of their work and their knowledge was respected. In 1921 Miss G S Brown was admitted as a Junior Member in Division C, subsequently became an Ordinary Member in 1924 and resigned from membership in 1928 – this record appears in the middle of the 1924 records, so it is possible that it is a clerical error and implies that the Division agreed her membership before admitting women had been agreed by the Committee.

More lady members were recorded in 1922: Miss E H Bedson and Miss S Glasscock were admitted as Ordinary Members in Division A. Given the rules at the time, this implies that Miss Brown had been working in a laboratory since at least 1916, and Miss Bedson and Miss Glasscock since 1917.

In 1924 Miss Bedson passed the examination in bacteriological technique and was therefore the first lady member to do so. The membership records for this period show that two of the ladies, Ann Wallace and Miss M Nash, held BSc degrees. This qualification is not recorded for any male PBLAA member – there is a Charles Otter with the letters L S B A after his name but it is not known what these stand for – and thus these ladies appear to be the first graduate members of the profession.

However, in 1938, Douglas Stanley, who started work as a medical laboratory technician in Sheffield in 1930, obtained a BSc (Hons) in chemistry from the University of London. He later qualified in medicine, became a pathologist and a founding Fellow of The Royal College of Pathologists. While a laboratory assistant, Stanley won the Junior Greenfield Prize and Medal and remained very proud of this throughout his life.

Between 1912 and 1941 a total of 2193 people were admitted to Junior, Ordinary or Associate membership, of which only 98 (4%) were ladies. All but one is recorded as 'Miss', and it was not until 1940 that a 'Mrs' Barbara

Pepper was recorded. This probably reflects the social mores and pressures of the time, when ladies were expected, if not required, to give up their careers upon marriage. The *Daily Herald* in October 1919 declared "No decent man would allow his wife to work… single women and widows should be given the work". In 1921, female civil servants passed a resolution asking that married women be banned from their jobs. As late as 1939, *The Monthly Bulletin* of the PBLAA carried an advertisement for a Woman Laboratory Assistant in the Ministry of Health Malaria Laboratory at Epsom. It stated that "normally candidates must be unmarried or widows and will be required to resign their appointment on marriage".

Chapter 5

Expansion, Examinations and Education

The Roaring Twenties: a decade of contradictions. Ten years of excess following the horrors of war; a period that saw a proliferation in the use of the radio and the very earliest developments of what was to become the ubiquitous television. In a room overlooking Praed Street in London, Alexander Fleming was the first man to observe penicillin in action and to appreciate its significance to medicine. Across the Atlantic, enactment of the 18th Amendment of the United States' Constitution resulted in the introduction, on 16 January 1920, of Prohibition – a measure not repealed until 1933.

Soon after the formation of the Association, Albert Norman realised that a certificate of competence, obtained by examination, would be vital if the status and abilities of laboratory assistants were to be recognised. Need for this was confirmed by the problems encountered with the War Office during the First World War over the recognition of members' abilities.

In January 1916, Norman was authorised to produce a preliminary scheme for such an examination. He started by reviewing the schemes already in place for a variety of other workers, including typists, inspectors of weights and measures, plumbers and midwives. When he had prepared the first draft it was sent to pathologists and senior members of the PBLAA for comment. Further drafts were produced and every detail was submitted to Professor German Sims Woodhead, who was, by this time, President, and serving in the Army in Tipperary. W A Mitchell recounts that while travelling to Ireland he would meet with Albert Norman in London, to discuss the drafts with him and have the difficulties explained before he showed them to the President. On his return, Mitchell would sometimes be at Norman's house in Wembley before 6.00 am to report progress. On other occasions, Norman, Chopping and McLean would meet his train at Euston to discuss developments. One valuable suggestion, which came from Dr Graham Smith, was for the appointment of officials who could assist and advise the examiners, and act as assessors during the practical examination.

Eventually, a subcommittee was appointed to produce the final draft of the scheme, which was adopted without the alteration of even a comma by the Association's committee. Albert Norman and W A Mitchell then presented the scheme to the committee of the Pathological Society at its meeting in Manchester. It was happy with it, in principle, and appointed Professors Boycott and Ledingham and Dr Murray to meet with Norman, Mitchell and McLean to discuss it in detail. When the scheme was approved this group became the Examining Council. In each district, two members of the Pathological Society were appointed as examiners, and one PBLAA member was appointed as an assessor. From the outset, the Association was assured that any member of the Pathological Society asked to be an examiner would give their whole-hearted support and would not accept payment. This was always honoured.

***

It was not until 5-6 July 1921 that the first examinations were held, in Edinburgh, Bristol, London, Liverpool and Manchester. The examinations consisted of a written paper of 90 minutes, a practical laboratory test of three hours, followed by an oral examination. Candidates were required to be at least 21 years old, have had five years' experience in an approved pathological and/or bacteriology laboratory, and have been a member of the PBLAA for at least six months. There were three main subjects: Bacteriological Technique, Pathological Technique and Pathological Museum Technique. In addition, there were a number of special subjects: Methods employed in the examination of urine and morbid secretions; Haematological and serological technique; Laboratory techniques of tropical medicine; Modelling in plaster, wax or papier-mâché; Articulation of bones; Photomicrography; Photography of laboratory and museum subjects, and other subjects approved by the Examining Council. Candidates could take the examination in more than one subject and paid an examination entrance fee of £2. 2s (£2.10p) for one subject, £1. 1s (£1. 5p) for each additional subject, or £3. 3s (£3. 15p) for all three. Special subjects were charged at 5s (£0. 25p). These fees became an important source of income for the PBLAA, particularly as the examiners received no fees.

Once the examination system was established it became clear that there was a number of mature and experienced men who had not sat a formal examination for many years, if ever, who might have been considered too senior to sit an examination to prove their abilities. As the lack of a certificate of competence could, in time, put these men at a disadvantage if they applied for a new post or promotion, an alternative was devised. During 1921 and 1922 these experienced men were given the opportunity to obtain certification on the basis of their experience. Applicants for this 'Certificate B' were required to have been members of the PBLAA for six months, be at least 30 years old, and have had 15 years' experience in an approved laboratory, no less than five years of this time being with one authority. The candidates were also expected to produce evidence acceptable to the Examining Council of their competence and suitability to hold the certificate. A fee of three guineas (£3.15) was charged. The first three certificates were issued to the Association's representatives on the Examining Council, Richard Muir, John McLean and Arthur Norman. Not all applications for Certificate B were successful, but over the two years it was awarded to 33 members.

A total of 35 candidates entered for the first examination: 16 were examined in all three sections, eight in two (bacteriology and pathology) and 11 in only one (one in bacteriology, 10 in museum technique), with eight being examined in special subjects. Successful candidates were awarded a certificate (Certificate A) signed by their examiners and by the President and Secretary.

In 1922 the number of entrants for the examination was much lower, the backlog having, to a great extent, been cleared in the first year. The examination continued in this format until 1929, when a much expanded syllabus was introduced. Pathological chemistry was added and museum technique was dropped; although it continued to be offered as a special subject. In this year only candidates who already held the Association's Certificate were allowed to enter for special subject examinations, and these became, in essence, a post-basic qualification.

***

In 1934 the length of the written examination was increased to 1 hour 45 minutes and new syllabuses were introduced. A new examination was introduced in 1937, for student members who had reached the age of 20 and had three years' experience in an approved laboratory. This became known as Part I and Certificate A became Part II. The Part I examination syllabus was based on an elementary knowledge of routine duties and methods common to the three major subjects of pathology: Histology, Bacteriology and Chemical Pathology. The first Part I examinations were held in November, in Birmingham, London, Manchester and Perth. The examination consisted of a written paper of 75 minutes, a practical of 150 minutes and a 15-minute oral. The written examination was set and marked by the committee and local examiners were responsible for the practical and oral portions.

Sixteen students entered this first Part I examination, and 10 passed. Successful candidates became Members of the PBLAA and were eligible to sit the Part II examination after a further two years' experience. This examination was held twice a year, in May and November (always on a Saturday), until May 1939. Owing to the outbreak of the Second World War, the November 1939 examination was postponed until 10 February 1940. During 1941, the call-up age for the armed forces was lowered and candidates aged 18 who had at least 18 months' experience were allowed to sit the Part I examination. However, when it was discovered that students who had been called up were allocated to laboratory duties, the normal age and experience requirements were reinstated.

Changes to the syllabus and arrangements were made over the years. The syllabus for the Intermediate examination issued in 1945 covered histology, bacteriology, chemical pathology and haematology. Candidates had to attempt questions in all subjects and obtain a pass mark of 60% in the practical as well as an aggregate 60% across all sections. Then, following discussions with and representations from the National Blood Transfusion Service, blood transfusion was added in 1957 as a separate subject. At the same time, candidates were allowed to 'opt out' of one of the five disciplines in the written, practical and oral components of the examination, although there was no requirement for it to be the same discipline in each section. The broad base of the examination was thus retained, but allowed the needs of those working in blood transfusion laboratories to be accommodated. A further adjustment occurred in 1959 when the written was increased to two papers and the practical and oral sections were held on separate days a month after the written examinations.

***

The Institute of Medical Laboratory Technology came into existence at the beginning of 1943 and took over responsibility for the examinations. The membership grades, together with the qualifications and the laboratory experience required, were redesignated. An Examining Board was established which comprised the President of the Institute and an equal number of representatives of the Pathological Society and Fellows of the Institute. The names of the examinations and the system of control were also changed. The Part I examination was renamed the Intermediate, with its own Examining Body consisting of Fellows of the Institute. The Part II examination became the Final examination, with an Examining Board comprising examiners (pathologists) and assessors (Fellows of the Institute).

The last PBLAA Part I examination was held on 12 September 1942 and the last Part II in July of the same year.

There is no doubt that the PBLAA examinations had a major impact on the profession. Many employers recognised the value of the certificate and made it a condition of employment for senior posts, and lack of it made advancement increasingly difficult.

The pattern of examinations continued as before, with Intermediate in the spring and autumn of each year, and the Final examinations on two consecutive days in July. Those who passed a Final examination were eligible to apply for entry to the class of Associate of the Institute of Medical Laboratory Technology, and were able to use the letters AIMLT after their name. Those with two Finals were eligible to apply for entry to the class of Fellows and use the designatory letters FIMLT.

The system for obtaining Fellowship of the Institute gave rise to complaints from those Associates working in specialist departments who had no opportunity, or indeed need, to gain the experience to pass a Final examination in another specialist subject. In response to this, an examination for Fellowship by Thesis was approved and made available from 1945. Application had to be made to the Examination Board for registration and approval of the subject of the thesis, together with evidence of the candidate's experience, and information about facilities for the research available to the candidate. It was expected that the thesis, of not less than 5000 words, would be largely technical, show evidence of originality and contribute new knowledge to the subject. Candidates were also subjected to an oral examination of their theses.

Later, in 1953, a further alternative route to Fellowship, by Dissertation and Examination, was introduced. This was aimed at those Associates who had neither the opportunity to change to another subject nor the facilities for practical research. This new Fellowship examination called for an "ordered and critical exposition of existing knowledge" presented as a formal bound report. Candidates also had to undergo written and oral examinations on their chosen subject.

The first Final examination in haematology and blood transfusion technique was held in December 1947, with the practical and oral papers being sat first. Only those who passed these papers were asked to sit the written examination in January 1948. Only two other Final examinations were added to the list: parasitology in 1950, and virology in 1960.

A request was made by the Royal College of Obstetricians and Gynaecologists for a Final in cytology, but this was rejected by the Institute. Similar requests were made for separate examinations in haematology and blood transfusion technique, but again this was not thought to be appropriate. The Final examinations were altered again in 1958 when the written section became two papers of two hours each (providing up to 60 marks), and a further paper of five 'short answer' questions (providing up to 40 marks). The practical and oral examinations continued as before. The title of the Pathological Technique examination was changed to Histopathological Technique.

From 1948 onwards the pass mark for the Final examination was 60% for the practical and an aggregate mark across all three sections of 60%. Any candidate who obtained an aggregate mark of less than 40% was not allowed to resit the examination the following year.

***

Up to 1964 the written papers were marked by members of the Examining Body (Final), but this was changed following recommendations made by Professor E T C Spooner. Subsequently, papers were marked by the examiners who were to mark the practical and oral sections, allowing them a better overall view of the candidate's abilities. Other changes were implemented at the same time. Assessors became examiners, a role previously entrusted only to pathologists, and all examiners were given equal status and would be paid a fee for their services (Council members who acted as examiners were not eligible for a fee, as they were directors of the company and not allowed to receive remuneration therefrom). For the first time in over 40 years, Fellows became examiners for their own profession and had control of those admitted to corporate membership.

Although the Council considered the possibility of holding the Intermediate examination overseas in 1944, and the government of India offered to make the Central Military Pathological Laboratory available for that purpose, it was not until 1956 that the first Intermediate examination was held overseas. It was conducted by Mr W H Valentine, a member of Council, the Examinations Board and the Examining Body (Intermediate), in Nigeria. Subsequently, examinations were held regularly in Nigeria and then in Ghana, Hong Kong, Kenya, Tanzania, Uganda and Mauritius, and many senior members of the profession acted as external examiners. Final examinations were never held outside the UK.

**

From the very beginning, education, training and the sharing of scientific, technical and management knowledge and skills were, and remain, the major role of the professional body. This followed naturally from one of its founding principles – "To assist in the general advancement of its members" – and from its motto *Disce ut proficias* (Learn, that you may improve).

The first meeting of members, for which records exist, was a meeting of Division D, held in Edinburgh on 6 December 1913. Following the important business of selecting the officers and representatives of the division, as well as matters affecting the formation of the Association and its rules, Richard Muir gave a lecture on malaria. At the next meeting, in January 1914, there was a talk, illustrated with specimens, on human and bovine tuberculosis, given by Mr W Watson; Mr Barr demonstrated the advantages of adding fuchsin to Dorset's egg medium, and Mr Muir gave a talk on filaria. This combination of discussion of local and national business with education became the normal pattern for division, region and branch meetings.

Division A (London) organised a series of lectures in 1922 and 1923, with topics including bacteriology technique, pathological technique, museum technique, the microscope, and post-mortem technique. The London, Manchester and Edinburgh divisions all advertised a series of lectures and demonstrations for the winter of 1927/28, London having an eight-week series aimed specifically at juniors, covering elementary bacteriology, pathology, cytology and museum technique. For the winter of 1928/29, the London, Birmingham, Liverpool and Manchester branches all advertised programmes of lectures, demonstrations and visits. Many, but not all, were given by members of the medical profession. In Birmingham there were two series, one aimed at 'seniors' and the other at 'juniors'. Cardiff held meetings on the first and third Thursdays of each month, but did not have an advertised programme. The Edinburgh branch arranged a programme of tuition for junior members in pathology conducted by Miss J C Muir, and in bacteriology technique by Mr A B Cheyne, both with the assistance of senior members of the branch. Mr T D Hamilton gave lectures and demonstrations on embryology to senior and junior members.

London broke new ground in 1930/31 by arranging a six-week 'Instructional Course in Biochemical Methods'. The following year, a 12-week course was arranged in Liverpool, which consisted of three weeks on the analysis of blood, four weeks on urine, two weeks on faeces and one week on gastric analysis. There was then a revision week and finally a practical examination. Inevitably, as many members worked in laboratories away from the larger centres, or were overseas or in the forces, not all were able to attend meetings of their division.

The role of the region and branch structure in education continues in this way, almost a century later, while 1957 saw the introduction of discipline-specific discussion groups. The London branch drew up terms of reference for such groups at its AGM that year. The first was a biochemistry group, which met in April, followed by haematology in August and bacteriology in September. One only has to look at *The Gazette* (now *The Biomedical Scientist*) each month to realise what a vast range of local, region and national meetings arranged by and for members and other interested parties took and continue to take place. This of course is now driven in no small way by the needs of continuing professional development (CPD).

***

The Laboratory Journal, and in time other publications, became an important vehicle through which information and education was provided. As well as publishing original papers, it included articles by members describing methods used in their laboratories, the answers to requests for information from members, and abstracts of papers published in other journals.

In the early years, the number of original articles was insufficient to fill the pages of each issue and the abstracts were included as a means to fill space. However, these became a valuable source of information at a time when access to a wide range of journals was difficult. These continued to be published until 1977.

Prominent members and other experts also contributed articles on important topics and technologies. Early articles included a series on 'Practical Media Making' by W A Mitchell and 'The Common Intestinal Protozoa of Man' by C M Weston, Director of Research in the Tropics to the Wellcome Bureau of Scientific Research. In 1916 there were articles on the theory and laboratory implications of the 'new' hydrogen ion theory as applied to bacteriology culture media, and the value of various indicators. Further articles on this subject were published in 1921. In the same year, a series of articles on clinical blood work (haematology) appeared, as did items on the care of laboratory animals and probably the first paper on 'laboratory management', written by John McLean, entitled 'Laboratory Administration'.

The original intention was to publish *The Laboratory Journal* four times a year, but this was not always possible due to the shortage of suitable articles and difficulties encountered during both world wars. No issues were published between 1918 and 1920 and thereafter only one or two issues a year were produced until 1937. As this was the only method of communication with the membership, naturally there was considerable dissatisfaction. It was suggested by Sidney Denyer and Frederick Chopping in 1933 that a second publication be produced to complement *The Laboratory*

Journal, which would remain as the Association's scientific publication. After investigation of the costs associated with producing a new publication and assessing the likely income from advertisers, they produced a rough copy and presented the proposal to Council. It gave support and appointed Denyer as Editor, aided by a production committee of H A Barker, C E Berry and F R Chopping.

The Monthly Bulletin was first published in April 1934 and contained items of general interest, including news from divisions, job vacancies, and movement of members. It also provided a forum for readers' questions, provided hints on technique, information on new equipment and references to publications. When, in January 1936, Sidney Denyer became General Secretary, Reginald Bromfield took over as Editor and continued in this role until 1950.

With the outbreak of war in 1939 it was decided to suspend publication of *The Laboratory Journal*; due to paper shortages and other difficulties, single issues of *The Laboratory Journal* were published in 1939, 1946, 1947 and 1950. *The Bulletin* continued to be published, albeit only bimonthly as an economy measure.

It is of great credit to Bromfield, who was based in London and despite the bombing and his duties as a fire watcher, that it never failed to be published. In March/April 1945 its name was changed to *The Bulletin of the Institute of Medical Laboratory Technology*. The final edition (Volume 15, No 6) was the November/December 1950 issue. The following year a new monthly 'house magazine', *The Gazette*, was launched. This was edited by S J Denyer, and Bromfield took on the role of Editor of the Journal – a post he held until 1966.

The contents of the Journal included Institute News, including examination results and election of new members; original articles; successful theses and the Greenfield and Sydney Mann prize essays; abstracts and references; laboratory notes; technical correspondence and book reviews. Gradually, news material transferred from the Journal to *The Gazette*, resulting in its transformation from a 'house journal' to a scientific journal of repute. However, *The Gazette* was not just a 'news sheet' but contained articles on issues relevant to the profession, and a vehicle for correspondence, and became an important method of keeping the membership informed of issues of the day. A further vital role, as seen by many of the membership, was the advertising of vacancies. In 1985 it became the *IMLS Gazette.*

The Journal was re-established as a quarterly publication in 1951 and renamed *The Journal of Medical Laboratory Technology*. It proved to be very popular and from 1964 the IMLT made arrangements for the Journal to be published by Academic Press. The title was shortened to *Medical Laboratory Technology* in 1967. Then, when the IMLT became the IMLS, the name was changed to reflect this and in 1976 it became *Medical Laboratory Sciences*.

Notwithstanding their official titles, they were known, and still are, as the Journal and the Gazette by the membership. Their function remains, as set out in an editorial note in the first issue of *The Journal* "to be of practical use to the membership in the various branches of pathological and bacteriological technique".

***

The role of the divisions and branches in courses for preparation for examinations and the wider education of members continued to expand. In December 1921, *The Laboratory Journal* published a report of an address given by Richard Muir to the London division in April 1920, when he set out the case for establishing courses of training for laboratory assistants. He described what was provided in his laboratory in Edinburgh – "A class of the members of the laboratory staff meets once or twice a week, from about 6.30 to 9.00 pm in the evening, to receive instruction in the form of a series of lectures and demonstrations". Following this, the London division started to plan how it might also offer a similar course, and in June 1922 there was a report congratulating this division on the success of its course of lectures and demonstrations, designed to meet the requirements of candidates for the Association's certificate. It was also reported that Liverpool and Manchester were hoping to start a similar scheme.

It became clear that courses aimed at those intending to sit the new Part 1 examination, which was to be introduced in 1937, were needed. In London, in 1936, a course and teaching syllabus was developed and introduced in six centres. This was an 18-week course of lectures, demonstrations and practical work, which concentrated heavily on technique and covered methods of dealing with glassware, sterilisation, laboratory apparatus and normal solutions, indicators, balances, adjustment of pH and simple urine tests, the preparation of culture media, making and examining cultures, staining methods, agglutination, the preparation of tissues for sectioning, use of the microtome, and cutting and staining sections by common routine methods. The fee for this course was 12s 6d (62.05p).

It is not clear how it proved possible for this branch of the Association to organise a course for an examination the syllabus for which had not been prepared. It seems likely that informal networking provided the necessary information. How widely this scheme was adopted outside London is not clear.

Although the PBLAA had decided that it was desirable that students should have reached a standard of education equivalent to the London University School Certificate, it was recognised that this was not always possible. In 1943, the newly formed IMLT Education Committee reiterated this advice and recommended that those students who did not possess this basic education should be encouraged to attend night school or undertake a correspondence course to obtain the appropriate level of basic education. It was also recommended that students should study two of the following subjects: physiology (to General Nursing Council standard), inorganic chemistry, biology or physics. The Institute approached employers and education authorities in the hope that these bodies would set up and run a scheme for technical instruction as well as basic sciences. It was not until 1945 that the Joint Committee on Salaries and Wages (Hospital Staffs) (JCS&W) – what may be seen as a precursor to the National Health Service Whitley Council (NHSWC) – required student technicians to have passed a recognised examination in general education (eg School Certificate). This body, which represented the major municipal, county and hospital associations in England and Wales, made recommendation after consulting medical experts and representatives of the IMLT.

This level of educational achievement then became a requirement for student membership of the IMLT. Later, in 1951, requirement for the School Certificate was replaced in England and Wales by O-level passes in English, Mathematics, Chemistry and one other science subject. With the subsequent adoption of the BTEC ONC qualification this was amended to English, Mathematics and two sciences. In 1956 it was agreed that graduates with one year's experience could enter a final examination, and that holders of an HNC in chemistry with five years' experience in a chemical pathology laboratory could be exempted from the written and practical parts of the final examination in chemical pathology. However, such people could only proceed to Fellowship by a thesis or dissertation in chemical pathology. It was also agreed that two A-levels, including chemistry, would give exemption from the Intermediate examination.

The general requirements of the Institute were formalised in Scotland from January 1946. All Scottish applications for student registration were required to possess the Junior Secondary Certificate and prior to sitting the Intermediate Examination should have successfully completed a further course in general and technical subjects at an approved Technical College, including English, Mathematics, Physics, Inorganic Chemistry, Physiology and Electricity & Magnetism. Further courses in chemistry were needed for those students taking pathological chemistry as a Final, and all students were required to attend Institute classes in bacteriology, haematology and pathology *(sic)*, haematology and pathological chemistry.

***

When the Institute of Medical Laboratory Technology was established in 1942 under the 1929 Companies Act, the objectives for which it was established included: "To advance the knowledge of practitioners of medical laboratory sciences by devising and imposing means of their qualifications by examinations either in theory or in practice, or in both, and to issue diplomas or certificates to the successful candidates. The Council shall supervise and approve professional examinations for admission to any class of membership and shall be satisfied as to the standard of education and training of candidates".

The IMLT Council set out to achieve these objectives by appointing an Educational subcommittee and through it the Board of Studies. The Board's tasks included the production of syllabuses for the examinations, and for tutors, and to set up and control both the examinations and tutorial systems. However, while the plans for training were being developed, the Edinburgh and Cardiff branches both submitted schemes for training students. The Edinburgh scheme was divided between the Herriot-Watt College (the local technical college) where basic sciences, physiology and mathematics were taught, and 'Institute work' which was carried out in the student's own laboratory and covered the basic laboratory techniques.

On first joining the pathology department of the Welsh National School of Medicine (WNSM), juniors were urged to continue their education through evening classes at the Technical College in subjects of value to their laboratory training, including chemistry, mathematics, physics, biology and a language. All fees were paid by WNSM and it was possible therefore for a student to obtain a science degree at its expense, and this had already happened on more than one occasion. Sheffield, in 1945, also set up its own syllabus and organised twice-weekly classes.

It would appear that it took longer to make the necessary arrangements than originally anticipated – after all the country was at war. Early in 1945 there was an announcement in *The Monthly Bulletin* (soon to become *The Gazette*) that it was hoped that the necessary arrangements for practical classes to start in October would soon be completed. In 1945, the Board of Studies produced detailed tutorial and course syllabuses for the Intermediate and Final examinations, as well as a course for the 'postgraduate' Certificate in Haematology. At this time, haematology was a relatively minor part of the work of a pathology laboratory and the course was confined to already qualified Fellows or Associates.

The Institute's scheme ensured that it maintained tight control over all aspects of the courses. It not only set the syllabuses and marked the examinations but appointed tutors and approved teaching premises. It achieved this through local tutorial committees, one for each centre or area.

These bodies, subject to the final approval of the Board of Studies, found the premises for courses, selected the tutors and, when necessary, demonstrators, enrolled the students, and collected and forwarded the fees (£2 2s 0d [£2.10p] per annum) to the Institute. Tutors had to be specialists in the subjects taught and either Fellows or Associates of the Institute. The Board made it quite clear that no unqualified person could be appointed to teach. Students, with the appropriate basic education, had to comply with the regulations on attendance. Poor attendance could lead to the student being removed from the course by the Board.

The courses for the Intermediate and Final examinations were of six terms of six weeks, three hours per week, over two years. The haematology course was 24 weeks. Tutors were expected to set and mark written questions and to conduct oral tests, which were designed to familiarise the student with the examination procedure. There were also recommendations about how isolated students could be helped by the tutor. Unfortunately the planned correspondence courses never materialised. The Board of Studies admitted that due mainly to the scarcity of suitable textbooks (and presumably the difficulties being experienced by students working in isolation in gaining access to them) this proved to be a more formidable task than at first envisaged.

During 1944, the Institute recognised the difficulties being experienced by students working in areas in which access to educational courses was difficult, and appointed Mr F W Jelks as student advisor. The aim of this role was to assist students in every way possible to sit the Intermediate examination and if necessary to reach the educational standard required for this examination. The first classes under the umbrella of the Institute were held in Belfast, Birmingham, Bristol, Edinburgh, Glasgow, Hull, Liverpool, London, Manchester, Oxford, Sheffield and the West Riding of Yorkshire.

In August 1946 the secretary, J M Signy, sent a letter to corresponding members of the Board of Studies, telling them that the Ministry of Education and the Ministry of Health had given approval for the establishment of classes in preparation for the Institute's examinations. The letter revealed that he had received 400–500 applications for enrolment in these classes. However, it would appear that the venues for these classes had yet to be decided as correspondents were asked, as a matter of extreme urgency, to recommend suitable premises.

Attached to the letter was a paper headed 'Supervision of Institute Classes'. It informed everyone that as the Institute's tutorial classes had now passed the experimental stage, supervision by the Institute was necessary to maintain standards. The paper set out, in some detail, the qualities required to be appointed as a tutor by the Board of Studies, the training of tutors, and the inspection of classes. Tutors and demonstrators were asked to complete an application form, which had to be countersigned by a Corresponding Member of the Board of Studies. The application also had to be signed by the director of the laboratory in which the tutor worked, in order to assist the Institute to gain approval for their appointment from the Ministry of Health.

The status of the Institute's qualifications was given a major boost when the JCS&W not only recommended the standard of education needed to be a student technician, but linked the other grades of technician to IMLT qualifications (ie junior technicians needed to have passed the Intermediate examination; technicians needed to have passed a Final examination, and a chief technician to have passed two Final examinations). These were far-reaching requirements as prior to this the Institute's qualifications had informal recognition only and were not a requirement for employment; indeed, it was not the only body which set qualifying examinations – both the Royal Army Medical Corps (RAMC) and the London County Council had their own. These recommendations, later adopted by the NHSWC, not only established the importance of IMLT qualifications for staff employed in hospitals and public health laboratories, but consolidated the position of the Institute as the sole provider of qualifications for those technicians employed in pathology.

Although the Institute approached the Ministry of Health and the Ministry of Education for cooperation and they promised assistance with the establishment of classes, very few held in 1946 were operated by a Local Education Authority (LEA). It was not until 1947, following a letter from Dr Burness of the Ministry of Education, that LEAs began to adopt the courses.

However, it took until 1958 for all Intermediate and Final courses to be held under the auspices of LEAs.

***

The 1944 Education Act introduced many far-reaching changes to the UK education system, but not all of its recommendations were implemented. The Act set out the intention that all young people, having left school at 15 years of age, could attend college for one day a week for 44 weeks a year until they were 18. Although the Institute pressed for this to be implemented, it was many years before day-release for Institute examinations was allowed. In late 1946, there was a meeting at the Ministry of Education with the aim of discussing the training of medical laboratory technicians. There were representatives of the Ministry of Education, Ministry of Health, the Scottish Health and Education departments, the PHLS, the Pathological Society, the British Postgraduate Medical School, the LCC Education Office, the Association of Clinical Pathologists and the Institute of Medical Laboratory Technology.

Dr Burness offered all possible help and wanted classes to be held during the day. The Ministry of Health representatives said that this would not be possible under the "present difficult circumstances" (ie staffing). In 1952–53, student technicians in Leicester attended a first-year Intermediate class in General Science Subjects on Thursday afternoons. This appears to be the first formal day-time provision of classes for the IMLT examinations and was probably unique. Even when, in 1954, a Ministry of Health Circular allowed hospitals to grant time off with pay and some expenses for attendance at classes in working hours, where no evening classes were available, night school continued to be the only method for study until March 1962. At this time, the Ministry of Health, suddenly and without warning, issued a circular that encouraged employers to allow student and junior technicians day-release with pay and expenses to attend courses leading to IMLT qualifications for up to six years. This was deemed sufficient time to allow a student to take and pass both the Intermediate and a Final and become 'qualified' and state registered.

Although the Institute, through the Joint Committee on Further

Education, had pressed for this for 15 years, the circular proved to be a surprise. In spite of this, a proposed course of study, incorporating basic science subjects, was prepared and published within three months of the announcement and the first day-release courses, for the Intermediate examination, were available for the 1962–63 academic year. By the end of 1967, day-time courses were available to virtually all students preparing for the Intermediate. In many centres, however, basic sciences were taught during the day and laboratory techniques were still taught in the evenings. This was because tutors for these subjects were drawn from local pathology departments, and many colleges lacked suitable laboratory premises. This pattern of day-release plus one evening continued after the introduction of the ONC and HNC qualification system.

***

At the end of the 1950s the IMLT examinations were well established and widely recognised as the appropriate qualification system for those working in pathology and related industries, and was essential for those employed in laboratories in the National Health Service. However, during the 1960s, various influential reports on education generally, on technical education and day-release appeared. These, and other developments, led the Council of the Institute to consider how the education and examination system for laboratory technicians should develop.

As early as 1948 there had been agreement in principle that the more basic sciences should be included in the courses and examinations. The Institute had also looked at the National Certificate system, but was concerned that it would lose control over the qualifying examinations. Nonetheless, as a result of the reports, it recognised the direction in which education was going and that there was a clear possibility that LEAs might not be willing or able to continue financing vocational courses, other than those schemes in which the government's education departments had a direct interest. These included National Certificates, but not courses run for private bodies such as the IMLT.

At a Council meeting in February 1961 it was resolved that education and training should be on "National Certificate lines", while retaining the Intermediate and Final examinations. When day-release for the IMLT became possible in 1962, the syllabuses devised by the Institute started to resemble those for national certificates. Discussions on how to respond to the growing pressures continued within the Institute and with relevant bodies. These culminated at a meeting of interested parties, when Jack Maitland-Edwards, Her Majesty's Inspector of Education with special responsibility for further and higher education in the public sector, raised the possibility, should the profession desire it, of a National Certificate scheme. This would be along the lines of the HNC in Chemistry and in Biology, which had been in existence since the 1920s. The Institute decided to pursue this suggestion and held many discussions with government ministries.

An Advisory Working Group was established in 1965 to look at the feasibility of national certificates. The group represented the Institute, the recently formed College of Pathologists, the Department of Education and Science, the Joint Committee for Ordinary National Certificates and Diplomas in Sciences, and the Scottish Education Department. It was generally agreed that this was the most advantageous route, but alternatives were discussed, including a degree course (rejected as impracticable at that time), block release or sandwich courses and full time OND and HND courses.

The first stage of the change was relatively straightforward. All national certificates in science had a common first stage, known as the Ordinary National Certificate in Sciences. There was a variant of the basic course designed for biologists and it was agreed that there would be a variant of medical laboratory technicians. This included the basic science subject syllabuses, to which were added a further syllabus that included bacteriology, haematology, histopathology, chemical pathology and blood transfusion from the Intermediate examination course. Two members of Council, Tom Lansley and Guy Pascoe, were appointed to represent the Institute on the Joint Committee for Ordinary National Certificates and Diplomas in Sciences. The first courses to follow this syllabus were introduced in September 1966.

The next stage, to produce a Higher National Certificate to the equivalent of a Final qualification, was more difficult. As well as the problem of producing a suitable syllabus, there were other hurdles to be overcome. The Registration Board of the Council for Professions Supplementary to Medicine needed to approve the changes and agree that the qualification was suitable for state registration. The Armed Forces used the IMLT qualifications and needed to be consulted. The scheme devised applied to England, Wales and Northern Ireland, but for Scotland a separate joint committee, consisting of the Institute and the Scottish Inspectorate, was needed. As the Republic of Ireland also used the Institute's examinations, its Department of Education needed to make alternative arrangements and set up a comparable joint committee.

The courses commenced in 1967, with retrospective approval being given to some two-year part-time courses intended to lead to the Final examination. The first HNCs were awarded in 1968. In Scotland, ONC courses were not introduced until 1967, and HNC not until 1969. Unlike the Scottish system, the England and Wales scheme permitted direct entry to HNC courses for holders of appropriate A-levels. In Scotland, all HNC students had to study the multidisciplinary ONC first. The ONC was accepted as suitable for ordinary membership of the IMLT, and HNC for admittance to the class of Associate. Holders of the HNC in Medical Laboratory Subjects were also eligible for state registration, but needed in addition to this three years' training in an approved laboratory. Those with A-levels who had bypassed ONC and gone straight into the two-year HNC course had a 'fallow' year. Many colleges took advantage of this by providing a pre-HNC bridging course during which the laboratory subjects were studied, thus providing a multidisciplinary background. Some colleges also offered conversion courses to established Fellows to teach them the basic sciences that had not been taught during Final courses, successful students being awarded HNC certificates.

Many senior and chief technicians had concerns about the apparent lack of uniformity from college to college and felt that HNC was not equivalent to a Final. However, comparison of the results obtained by those who sat both examinations in 1968 and 1969 showed that the results were similar.

With the adoption of the National Certificate system of education and qualification, it was decided to phase out the Intermediate and Final examinations. The last Intermediate was held in the autumn of 1970 and the last Final in 1975. After this time the Institute changed its function from that of a qualifying body to a professional one. It is true to say that a large proportion of the membership viewed this with regret, many taking the view that "we had lost control of our profession and placed it in the hands of the educationalists". Despite this, many members of the profession went into teaching, and the aphorism 'them that can, do; those that can't, teach' being rather unfairly applied to them.

There was also considerable concern about the ability of full-time lecturers to keep up to date with current laboratory methods and practice. These concerns were misplaced and unfair, as in almost all cases the pathology laboratory sciences continued to be taught by the same laboratory-based tutors who had run and taught night classes. The Institute and its members were closely involved with the colleges providing the courses, not only approving the syllabuses but providing most, if not all, teaching of what were to become known as biomedical sciences. As they also set and marked the examinations in these subjects, it is arguable that they were more closely involved with qualification standards than under the previous system. Nonetheless, there was a great deal of suspicion and misunderstanding of both the purpose and content of the ONC and HNC system.

A letter published in *The Gazette* in 1966, from a Fellow who was also a full-time lecturer in medical laboratory science, pointed out that "the course was based on the assumption that the very high standard of technical competence…is best achieved in the laboratory under the guidance of experienced and qualified laboratory staff"; whereas the role of the colleges was to teach the basic sciences so that technicians had a better understanding of the principles underlying methods used then and in the future. Possibly the most contentious subject was 'general studies'. Senior laboratory staff strongly resented their staff having time off (as they saw it) to study subjects which, in their view, had no direct relevance to laboratory work. They were not convinced by the 'mind broadening' aspect of this requirement.

Although only Associateship was needed to become state registered (once the Final examinations had stopped, HNC became the normal qualification for registration and it was not necessary to join the Institute), and, within the NHS, to be promoted to technician, Fellowship was needed for promotion to the higher grades of technician in the NHS. This, coupled with the increasing specialisation seen in pathology laboratories (more people were working in single-discipline departments rather than in multidisciplinary laboratories) meant that an alternative route to Fellowship was needed before Final examinations were phased out. Other routes had been considered in the past; a meeting of examiners (pathologists) in 1955 proposed that Fellowship should consist of a more advanced examination in the same subject as that required for Associateship, but this was rejected because the thesis or dissertation route was thought to be a satisfactory alternative. It became obvious that a few Associates a year submitted either a thesis or dissertation. In January 1964, Council approved an Advanced Examination for Fellowship, which was to be assessed at a higher level in the subject in which the candidate qualified as an Associate. As the examination system was included in the Articles of Association, a special resolution to replace examination by dissertation with examination by dissertation or advanced examination was put to the Annual General Meeting held in Leeds later that year. It was rejected. The following year, Council put a resolution to the AGM to remove the examination systems from the Articles of Association. This was passed, as was a resolution establishing what became known as the Special Examination for Fellowship.

The new examination was introduced in 1966. It comprised three written papers, one being an essay of at least 1000 words, the candidate being given a choice of two topics on which to write. In addition, there was a short essay paper and a multiple-choice paper. Those reaching a minimum mark in the written section were invited to attend a searching and extended oral examination. The disappointing pass rate of 38% was attributed to candidates not being able to attend a two-year course in preparation for the examination. The following year the pass rate was even lower, at 23.5%. The examiners indicated that the poor results were due to the failure of candidates to realise that the level of knowledge required was much higher than that needed for Associateship. Eventually the Special Examination became the principal route to Fellowship and as a result the dissertation was phased out in 1968 and the Final examination in 1975. Not many members entered for the Special Examination in Parasitology and it was discontinued in December 1972.

There were no formal courses for the Special but many centres offered evening classes designed to prepare candidates for the examination. In 1974 the Institute decided that properly organised courses were needed, and it suggested that there should be mandatory attendance at a further education course – a minimum of 250 hours, over two years. In addition, there would be continuing assessment, based on at least 100 hours home work, as well as a project report based on a practical investigation, again expected to take at least 100 hours. Marks for the project and the course assessment counted for 30% of the marks.

The Institute set four written papers, three of which were essay style designed to test the depth and range of the candidate's ability to express opinions based on sound data and reasoning, knowledge of academic principles and vocational applications of the subject. The fourth was a multiple-choice paper comprising 80 five-choice questions.

The new examination was launched in 1977, but only 15 colleges offered approved courses by the end of that year.

Transition arrangements were made during which course attendance was not necessary; however, the pass rate among those who attended approved courses was twice that of those who did not. Furthermore, it is interesting to note that entrants with a science degree had a higher pass rate than those with HNC, who in turn did better than those who passed the Institute's Final examination.

***

Over the years several attempts were made to establish a lending and reference library. The 1920 PBLAA constitution had this as one of its objectives. Although Dr Carnegie Dickson made a donation for the purchase of technical books, the logistical difficulties of housing and administering proved to be insurmountable. There was a further attempt in 1926 when it was suggested that an Association library be formed using the library of the Liverpool branch as a nucleus. There is no record of the Liverpool branch's response to this proposal, but the library was not established. However, on 1 January 1928 the Association established a Lending Library scheme, which allowed members to borrow books from the H K Lewis Circulating Library, situated in Gower Street, London. In the annual report for 1928 it was recorded that a total of 50 books had been borrowed in the first six months of the service, and this was considered by the Committee "to be a boon to the members who have taken advantage of it". In 1944 a further attempt was made. The annual report for that year stated that "it is intended to establish an Institute library and gifts of books would be welcome". Initially, only seven books were received and over the next seven years further donations were made.

In 1962, Mr John R Mercer presented a detailed proposal for an Institute library to a meeting of the London branch. Mr Richard J Lavington, the General Secretary of the Institute, who was at the meeting, took John Mercer's proposal to the July meeting of Council. The proposal to establish a reference library was approved and John Mercer was appointed Honorary Librarian. The Librarian, through donations and purchases, has established a unique collection of textbooks on pathology laboratory technique and associated subjects. The library also holds the collection of Fellowship theses and dissertations as well as a complete set of *Journal*, *Bulletin* and *Gazette*, and many other books and documents of historical importance.

***

Initial membership of the Association was small, although around 120 assistants expressed interest in joining in 1912, but of the 117 members recorded at the end of 1912 only 95 were recorded as members in 1913. Increase in membership was slow but steady. In 1914, at the outbreak of the First World War, there were 143 members based in the UK plus 38 overseas members, of whom 27 were in Sydney, Australia. In 1915 this rose to 155 plus 55 overseas members, including the Australian membership of 41, nine of these being based in Melbourne. When the Association resumed activities in

1920, UK membership stood at 163. The majority, 142, of these members were so-called seniors, and the remaining juniors. This slow but steady rise continued and at the end of the decade the number of members had reached just under 600. In addition, there were two Life Members, 20 Honorary Members and eight Associate members. A membership of 1000 was not reached until 1936 and was at around this level when normal life again was interrupted by the outbreak of the Second World War. When hostilities ceased in 1945 the membership at the end of that year was around 1500. The changes brought about by the formation of the National Health Service in 1948, together with an increasing requirement for laboratory investigations, resulted in a rapid increase in both the number of laboratories and the number of laboratory technicians.

By the time the Institute celebrated its Golden Jubilee, in 1962, membership stood at over 9000. An increasing membership brought about alterations to the division and branch structure. The original four divisions increased to five by adding one for overseas members. This structure remained in place until the formation of the IMLT in 1943, when divisions became regions. In 1946 there were six regions: London and South Eastern, with a membership of approximately 1000; South Western, 100; Midland, 160; Northern, 350; Scottish, 220; and Irish, 50. Regional representation did not include overseas members. In the late 1930s there were about a dozen branches, some more active than others. In 1946 this had risen to 22 and by 1975 had increased to 45 with three sub-branches. As will be seen elsewhere, not only did the organisation of the membership increase in complexity but so too did the administrative and committee structure of the Institute.

Chapter 6

Conferences and Triennials

In the almost 70 years that elapsed between the discovery of penicillin in 1928 and the end of Margaret Thatcher's tenure as Prime Minister in the early years of the 1990s, antibiotic therapy proved first to be a therapeutic panacea and subsequently to be a potential weakness in the medical armamentarium. The ability of single-celled microorganisms to develop resistance to powerful chemotherapeutic agents was unexpected yet it became evident soon after their introduction. Despite this, the so-called antibiotic age has seen significant advances in medicine that otherwise might not have been possible.

The Association had always planned to hold national conferences, an aspiration consistent with the founding principle of assisting with general advancement of its members and with the Association's motto. In the report of the meeting of the Provisional Committee in 1912, both Professor Lorrain Smith and John McLean recognised the value of holding such meetings and hoped that they would become a normal part of the Association's activities. They hoped that such meetings would facilitate the formal and informal exchange of ideas and practices, help develop contacts and improve the corporate identity of the Association and its members – now referred to as 'networking'.

In 1921 the President, Sir German Sims Woodhead, suggested that it would be good if the Association could hold regular meetings for exhibitions and discussions of laboratory matters. But it took 12 years from its foundation before the Association felt it was mature enough to hold its first Conference. This was held in the Department of Pathology in the University of Edinburgh, viewed by many as the cradle of the Association.

***

The Edinburgh Conference (1–5 September 1924) was planned and hosted by the members of Division D. It was well attended; 54 members (about 16% of the UK membership) and 24 visitors signed the attendance book (the attendance book is numbered and the last signature was No 64, but Nos 40–49 are missing). However, several people who did not sign the register appear in the official Conference photograph, and as there is a gap in the sequence of numbers in the register, there were probably more attendees than shown in the records. Most of those who attended were from Scotland, 11 travelled from London and there were several from other parts of England and Wales. One member, Mr H Bailey, travelled from Cape Town, South Africa, and two visitors were from India – Major J A Cruickshank of the Indian Medical Service, and S Ramallissman. All but one of the ladies who attended were visitors, the exception being Miss J C Muir from Edinburgh, who attended as a member in her own right.

How the conference was funded is not totally clear. An allocation of £10 was made from Association funds and at a meeting of members of Division D a total of £20.19s.0d (£20 95p) was promised by those present. A notice in the March 1924 issue of *The Laboratory Journal* asked members who planned to attend to inform the Secretary as soon as possible as it would "greatly assist the Committee in arranging for travelling and estimate the approximate cost per individual". No mention is made of a Conference fee or a charge for visitors or accompanying wives etc. However, charges were made for excursions and sightseeing tours. There was a full scientific and social programme.

The Conference was opened by the Vice President, Thomas D Hamilton, who after his opening welcome gave a lantern-slide lecture on the History of Edinburgh. This was followed by two films, one on the prevention of malaria, the other on hookworms. Nearly all of the presentations and demonstrations were given by members of the Association and covered several disciplines: Virology – the Diagnosis of Rabies, by Albert Norman; Museum technique – *passe-partout* binding and maceration of bones; Bacteriology – the diagnosis of diphtheria, and the chromogenic mycobacteria; Histology – the large Cambridge Microtome, and paraffin embedding apparatus; Management – a discussion on laboratory economics. There were also talks by two veterinary surgeons, one on the recently discovered 'bacteriophage phenomenon', the other on various infections of animals.

During the first four days there were demonstrations by members on laboratory methods, including those relating to tropical diseases. At the end of each afternoon, there were visits and tours of places of interest in and around Edinburgh. Members were invited to bring "their lady friends" to these and to the Monday morning session. The only event on Friday was the conference dinner. Those attending were advised that "Evening Dress is not desirable". Following a six-course meal, which included Fried Sole with Toastit Tatties and Roastit Hen with Tatties (Hale or Champit), the President, Professor A E Boycott FRS, proposed a toast to 'The King', and Albert Norman was presented with the first Sims Woodhead Medal. The President and members from the south had to leave before the end of proceedings to catch the mail train to London (an overnight express).

The Conference was fully reported in the July 1925 issue of *The Laboratory Journal*. There was general agreement that the first Conference was a great success and should become a regular event, as had been suggested by German Sims Woodhead (by this time deceased).

***

In an article extolling the advantages and attractions of Cambridge as a Conference centre, W A Mitchell assured those members planning to attend the meeting (22–26 August 1927) that the Cambridge branch would do its best to maintain the high standard set by the Edinburgh branch.

The conference was opened by The Vice-Chancellor of Cambridge University. In his address he expressed the view that the existence of the Association indicated that the members "were not content to be just competent and efficient officials; they wanted to increase scientific knowledge". He greatly admired that, in keeping with the highest standards of their scientific departments, those present should spend part of their holiday attending a conference of this kind. He also recounted an occasion when Professor Sims Woodhead, a man who loathed alcohol, drank a bottle of whisky to test the effect on his temperature.

Following the Vice-Chancellor's address, Mr W A Mitchell gave a lantern-slide lecture on Cambridge. Following the Official Photograph there was a Garden Party in the Fellows' Garden of Downing College, a Cricket Match, a Tennis Tournament and Tea in the College Hall. The Conference proper started on the Tuesday morning and during this and the next two mornings there were lectures and demonstrations on plague and smallpox vaccine manufacture; tissue culture of a wide range of tissues including a pulsating heart culture; bacterial identification; parasitology; a visit to the Institute of Animal Pathology and various museum and illustration techniques.

More people attended this conference than the one in Edinburgh. Altogether, 110 signed the attendance register; 67 members and 43 visitors. There was also an international flavour to the meeting with speakers from South Georgia, the Gold Coast (Ghana) and Uganda. Mr A E P Grimmo had travelled from Shanghai, a distance of some 11,000 miles, to attend the

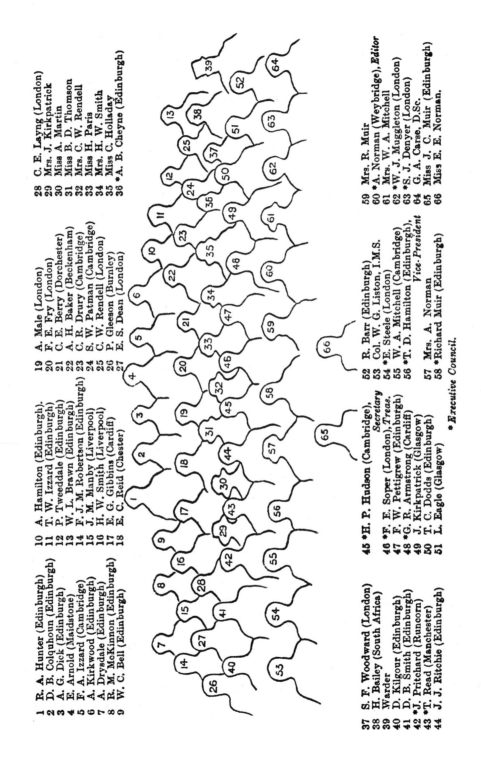

1 R. A. Hunter (Edinburgh)
2 D. B. Colquhoun (Edinburgh)
3 A. G. Dick (Edinburgh)
4 E. Arnold (Maidstone)
5 F. A. Izzard (Cambridge)
6 A. Kirkwood (Edinburgh)
7 A. Drysdale (Edinburgh)
8 R. M. McKinnon (Edinburgh)
9 W. C. Bell (Edinburgh)

10 A. Hamilton (Edinburgh).
11 T. W. Izzard (Edinburgh)
12 P. Tweeddale (Edinburgh)
13 W. L. Brawn (Edinburgh)
14 F. J. M. Robertson (Edinburgh)
15 J. M. Manby (Liverpool)
16 H. W. Smith (Liverpool)
17 E. G. Gibbins (Cardiff)
18 E. C. Reid (Chester)

19 A. Male (London)
20 F. E. Fry (London)
21 C. E. Berry (Dorchester)
22 A. H. Baker (Beckenham)
23 C. R. Drury (Cambridge)
24 S. W. Patman (Cambridge)
25 C. W. Rendell (London)
26 P. Gleeson (Burnley)
27 E. S. Dean (London)

28 C. E. Layng (London)
29 Mrs. J. Kirkpatrick
30 Miss A. Martin
31 Miss B. D. Thomson
32 Mrs. C. W. Rendell
33 Miss H. Paris
34 Mrs. H. W. Smith
35 Miss C. Holladay
36 *A. B. Cheyne (Edinburgh)

37 S. F. Woodward (London)
38 H. Bailey (South Africa)
39 Warder
40 D. Kilgour (Edinburgh)
41 D. B. Smith (Edinburgh)
42 *J. Pritchard (Runcorn)
43 *T. Read (Manchester)
44 J. J. Ritchie (Edinburgh)

45 *H. P. Hudson (Cambridge), *Secretary*
46 *F. E. Soper (London), *Treas.*
47 F. W. Pettigrew (Edinburgh)
48 *G. R. Armstrong (Cardiff)
49 J. Kirkpatrick (Glasgow)
50 T. C. Dodds (Edinburgh)
51 L. Eagle (Glasgow)

52 R. Barr (Edinburgh)
53 Col. W. G. Liston, I.M.S.
54 *E. Steele (London)
55 W. A. Mitchell (Cambridge)
56 *T. D. Hamilton (Edinburgh), *Vice-President*

57 Mrs. A. Norman
58 *Richard Muir (Edinburgh)

59 Mrs. R. Muir
60 *A. Norman (Weybridge), *Editor*
61 Mrs. W. A. Mitchell
62 *W. J. Muggleton (London)
63 *S. J. Denyer (London)
64 G. A. Carse, D.Sc.
65 Miss J. C. Muir (Edinburgh)
66 Miss E. E. Norman.

Executive Council.

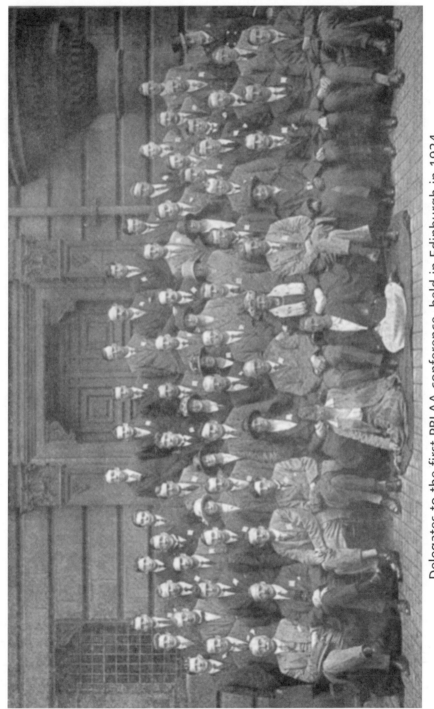

Delegates to the first PBLAA conference, held in Edinburgh in 1924

Conference and take his examinations. Good wishes for a successful Conference were received from members in Uganda, Kenya and the Gold Coast. The Medical Sciences Laboratory Assistants' Association of Australia hoped that, in the not too distant future, there might be an Empire or even an International Conference.

The Cambridge organising committee not only built on the success of the Edinburgh Conference but made innovations of their own, including a Reception Room, where impromptu parties and dances were held. They also introduced a Ladies' Committee, members of which prepared and served refreshments in the mornings and evenings. It was hoped that both the Reception Room and the Ladies' Committee would become an important feature at future conferences.

Those who were unable to attend the Conference were not forgotten as again the editor of *The Laboratory Journal* ensured the papers read at the meeting were published, as was an overview of the other activities. The conference was also reported extensively in both the *Cambridge Daily News* and *The Cambridge Chronicle and University Journal*.

Once again, it is not clear how the costs of the conference were covered. Council felt that it was too much to expect Cambridge members to cover the costs of entertaining their colleagues and any incidental expenses, although this was paid by the Scottish members at the first conference. Therefore, Council allocated a sum not exceeding £50 for this purpose. In the event, the Garden Party was financed by Members of the Cambridge Department of Pathology, and the Scottish members were the guests of the London members at the Conference dinner, and only £27 6s 1d (£27.30) was spent from this allocation.

***

The arrangements for the third Conference, in Manchester (25–29 August 1930), were much as before, with of course innovations and expansion. On the scientific side there were many more exhibits and demonstrations and a good range of papers on various topics. The Thursday morning session included an open discussion, led by John McLean and Frederick Chopping, on the training of juniors. The excursions and visits were both of a cultural and educational nature. Separate excursions were organised for ladies, including a visit to a bakery and to Liverpool, and there were tours of the surrounding area for all delegates.

For the first time a Conference Handbook was produced. This contained not only useful information about the meeting and Manchester but also advertisements for laboratory supplies and for local hotels and places of interest. As there is no mention of the cost of the handbook in the accounts, it must be assumed that it was financed through the charge made for these adverts. The total cost of the conference was £58 7s 9d (£58.40), of which £50 came from central funds. The number of delegates rose to 77 but as a percentage of the membership this was lower than the two previous conferences.

The proceedings were reported in *The Laboratory Journal* and the local press (*The Manchester Guardian*). Reports in *Nature* and the *British Medical Journal* both referred to the meeting as the third 'triennial' conference – the first time this descriptive phrase was used. In later years the Conference was more often known as the 'Triennial'. However, a national newspaper, the *Daily Express*, was only interested in the members' 'scientific' verdict on Manchester's women and Manchester's weather!

***

The London Conference (21–26 August 1933), held in the London School of Hygiene and Tropical Medicine, was notable for a number of 'firsts'. It was the first time 'Triennial Conference' was used in the title; it was the first Conference to be opened by the President, Dr J A Murray FRS; the first to have what was termed a 'Trades Show'; and the first to have a discussion on Association activities. The events, set out in the Conference Handbook and separate programme, followed the well-established mixture of scientific papers, demonstrations, exhibits and social events. Not all visits were for sightseeing, as delegates had the opportunity to visit the laboratories and farm of the Express Dairy Company and the National Institute for Scientific Research. Two new social events were introduced at this gathering: a conversazione, the expenses of which were borne by Division A, and a post-conference tour on the Saturday after the conference.

The opening address by the President contained remarkably prescient and far-sighted predictions. He believed that "standardisation of methods will ultimately permit delegation of much of the routine work at present reserved to fully qualified members of the medical profession (there was at that time no qualifying examination in any field of pathology for the medical profession, but there was for pathology laboratory assistants – Ed), to properly qualified technical assistants and this implies an obligatory system of certification superseding the voluntary certification established by the Association". Predictions which, although taking many years to be fulfilled, came true and were exceeded.

The discussion of Association activities inevitably brought both praise and complaints. There were criticisms of the irregular appearance of *The Laboratory Journal*, and the low examination pass rate. There were also complaints about poor communication by Council with the members. Members were particularly upset that they had not been made aware of discussions about a possible change to the name of the Association. A subcommittee had been set up to consider this and three of the names being considered included the title Technician. As will be seen, the work of this subcommittee led eventually to the Institute of Medical Laboratory Technology. Nevertheless, the conference was judged by the 94 members who attended from the UK and abroad to be a great success.

***

The fifth Triennial Conference, in Edinburgh (24–29 August 1936), was the last held under the auspices of the PBLAA. The programme for this conference was much as before but with a more complex content. In his opening address, the President, Professor J McIntosh, drew attention to the rapid developments that were being made in medical science and felt it was the duty of the Association to keep abreast of the times.

As the demand for investigations had increased 10-fold in the previous 20 years, he said he was sure that this increase would continue and create new problems for hospitals, particularly teaching hospitals, and that there was likely to be a greater demand for laboratory assistants to carry out the work in hospitals. Professor McIntosh warned laboratory workers not to become mere technicians! He felt that they had a broader outlook and could acquire knowledge outside their own particular branch.

Both the President's address and some of the papers were reported in the Edinburgh newspapers. One Conference paper reported highlighted the dangers of falling into the Thames and the risks of contracting *Leptospira icterohaemorrhagiae*. Another report was on a paper given by Mr A Walters of the Albert Dock Hospital (a hospital situated near the London docks which specialised in the care of merchant seamen) on the problems of carriers of enteric fever and the risks they posed to contacts. It is interesting that *The Edinburgh Evening News* used the headline 'A hand shake may carry infection'; now, over 70 years later, similar headlines still appear in newspapers, but they now refer to methicillin-resistant *Staphylococcus aureus* (MRSA) and similar microorganisms. *Plus ça change…!*

Over 100 members attended the Conference, which represented about 10% the membership at that time. One wonders whether more would have attended had they known that the discussion about future activities of the Association would, as will be seen elsewhere in the book, prove to have a major impact on the future, not only of the Association but also the profession at large. The meeting was chaired by Mr A B Cheyne – the Vice President – and also on the platform were Albert Norman (Secretary to the Examining Council) and Sidney Denyer (General Secretary). The discussion was opened by Mr Sydney Laws, who was on leave from Uganda. He gave a clear analysis of the possibilities for the future development of the Association. These were either to seek a Royal Charter or to become a company limited by guarantee. His conclusion and advice was for the PBLAA to become a company limited by guarantee, and he further proposed that it become an institute and included the words Laboratory Technicians in its title. He went on to propose grades of membership based on examination, entry to which would be based on periods of training in 'approved' laboratories.

After wide-ranging discussion it was agreed to plan for the formation of a company and an institute. During the discussion, various alternative titles to the PBLAA were suggested, including Institute of Technical Pathologists and Bacteriologists; …Medical Technicians and …Medical Laboratory Technicians. However, many felt that the terms 'pathologist' and 'bacteriologist' were inaccurate and limiting. After assurances that those working in the veterinary field would not be excluded, the title Institute of Medical Laboratory Technicians found favour with many of those present. The other suggestion made by Laws, to register with the National Register of Medical Auxiliary Services, the controlling interest of which lay with the British Medical Association, was rejected.

A further discussion was held on the value of obtaining the Association's certificate. It transpired that recognition of the certificate by employers was irregular. It was evident that while considerable advances had been made by the Association on behalf of its members, there was still a long way to go in some areas – some employers gave staff increases in pay when they obtained the qualification, while others made possession of the certificate a condition of employment, and it was essential for Colonial Office overseas appointments.

However, Birmingham took no notice of the certificate as the authorities there did not recognise the Association. Other municipal employers, such as the London County Council, took a different view, and gave their staff working in the Mental Hospital Service laboratories a salary increase of £13 per annum. However, the University of Edinburgh classed technical staff with unskilled workers in its non-contributory pension scheme.

A meeting was planned for 1939 but, as there were soon to be fundamental changes to the constitution of the Association, it was decided not to hold a Conference. It had been hoped to hold a meeting in 1940, but the onset of war meant that none were held until 1949.

***

There had been many significant changes during the 13 years since the last Conference. The most important of which were PBLAA was now the Institute of Medical Laboratory Technology (IMLT) and the National Health Service had come into being.

The formal proceedings of the Oxford Conference (24-29 July 1949) were opened by Professor A D Gardner (Regis Professor of Medicine in the University of Oxford). He spoke of the changes and developments he had seen during the 40 years since he first worked in a laboratory as a medical student. Not only had the scope of a technician's work expanded but their skill and status had increased, due in no small part to the efforts of the PBLAA. He went on to talk about the high cost of hospital services, pointing out that hospitals were heavily in debt when the NHS was formed, and costs continued to rise. In 1930 the average cost per patient was £3, which by 1949 was £12. He noted that during his lifetime there had been (in his words) "a gradual invasion of laboratories by women". Although, quite probably, some of the senior members present at this conference had opposed the change, few, he thought, "would now maintain that women as a whole had not made good in the laboratory. Moreover, it was convenient to have a good proportion of junior posts filled by girls, because they soon thinned out by marriage and so prevented congestion in the higher ranks". He was, however, glad to see that boys were no longer employed in dead-end jobs.

As before there was a full programme of scientific papers, demonstrations and exhibits, including a trade exhibition, on Thursday and Friday, as well as a variety of receptions, tours, visits and the Conference dinner. Most of those attending were housed in Keble College which enhanced the corporate feeling and proved to be a very popular innovation. At the dinner, a portrait of Albert Norman was presented to the Institute, as was a bronze plaque on which to record the names of the recipients of the Sims Woodhead Medal. Both now hang in the Council chamber of the Institute at Coldbath Square.

An innovation for this Conference saw the Annual General Meeting of the Institute held during the week. A discussion entitled 'The Institute, the Technologist and the Future' was chaired by Albert Norman. Mr W H Valentine opened the discussion, and after giving a résumé of the history of the Association and Institute, he said that "whereas technicians were formerly thought of a scattered assortment of individuals, they are now thought of as a body of workers". He felt that this cohesion was due to the formation of the professional body.

With over 2000 members and around 1660 student members, he felt that the Institute would continue to have considerable influence in the future. In support of this, he cited the advice it was able to give in the formulation of national pay scales for those employed in the NHS (as the Institute was not a trades union, it could not sit on the staff-side of the Whitley Council, but was able to act as an advisor). Other points raised by Mr Valentine included recognition of the more organised education system, while, during the discussion, members raised difficulties experienced with the employment of science graduates and problems with developing and conducting examinations.

***

The first six Conferences have been described in some detail as they established the format for the 'Triennial'. In essence, the Conferences held between 1952 and 1992 followed the same format; a mixture of lectures, exhibitions and demonstrations balanced with plenty of time for visits to places of interest and other social activities. It is important to remember that members attending the early meetings usually did so in their time and at their own expense. It was many years before employers gave study leave with expenses for attending such meetings. So, Conference was part education and part holiday.

Many of the men attending brought their wives and parts of the social programme were aimed at this group. Many of these activities would now be thought of as sexist and patronising, but they reflected the social attitudes of the time. Gradually, the balance between the holiday and educational aspects of Conference changed and, while the social networking aspects of the meetings remained important, the educational content grew, as did the reputation of the Triennial as a scientific meeting.

This rise in importance grew alongside the massive expansion of pathology and the increase in Institute membership. From 1949 until the last Conference in 1992 the meetings were held in universities during the summer vacation. This had the double advantage of providing facilities for the lectures and accommodation for the delegates on one site.

The Opening Ceremony was always held on the Monday morning, although gradually the formal events commenced on Sunday with a service of dedication. The Opening Ceremony took the same general format, and included an address of welcome, usually by the Vice-Chancellor of the university or someone of similar standing. After a reply by the Institute President, there was a speech from an important politician or person of significance in healthcare or science.

The scientific programme started on Tuesday and finished on Friday. In the early years there was only one series of talks per morning, the afternoon being devoted to tours and visits. In 1962 there were sufficient papers for there to be parallel sessions. In 1965 this increased to three simultaneous lecture sessions and in 1980 this rose to four. A further innovation in 1962 was the introduction of discipline-specific discussion group meetings. These were held in the afternoon and proved to be very popular.

While visits of general interest and sightseeing continued to be offered, the balance moved towards those more relevant to science and pathology. These included tours of specialist laboratories, manufacturer's premises and similar venues, occasionally including a local brewery or distillery, which would, of course, be of interest to microbiologists and chemists. The Bristol Conference in 1958 hosted an open meeting of the International Association of Medical Laboratory Technologists and a special programme of visits was arranged for the overseas visitors.

The 'trade show' first became a feature of Conference in 1933, when 13 companies, all approved by the organising committee, exhibited a range of laboratory equipment and materials. This proved to be a popular innovation and grew to be a major feature of subsequent conferences. Although only two companies exhibited in 1936, after the war the number of exhibitors rose steadily and in 1980 over 100 companies took stands at the Belfast Conference, and many others placed advertisements in the Conference literature. The importance of the Triennial to manufacturers and suppliers was shown by many of them choosing to launch new products at the meeting.

Some also sponsored symposia, outside the main meeting, centred on applications related to their equipment or reagents.

***

It was problems with the trade show in 1992 in Liverpool that exposed the underlying weakness in the way the Triennial was organised. The meetings had been planned and operated, in the main, by a committee formed by members of the local Institute branch and members of Council, together with administrative assistance from staff at the Institute's headquarters. By 1992 it had become clear that the size and complexity of the Triennial required more time and expertise than could be provided by this group.

The problems, however, were not solely about administration. Both the membership and the commercial companies criticised the venue. The trade show was housed in a marquee on a site distant from the lecture theatres, making it difficult for delegates to visit. In addition, the opening of the trade show was marred by a lack of electricity. The situation was not helped by the weather, as heavy rain made the grass on which the marquee stood soft and muddy. Stands started to sink into the soft ground and some exhibitors had to resort to buying Wellington boots to keep their feet dry.

The organisation had been subcontracted to what were believed to be appropriate and experienced subcontractors; however, they failed to live up to expectations and steps were taken to obtain compensation and damages. Many of the exhibitors made their dissatisfaction very clear and threatened to boycott future Triennial conferences and hold their own meeting in competition with the Triennial.

Problems with the Liverpool Triennial were exacerbated by the fact that the lectures were held in the city centre campus while the accommodation was situated on the outskirts of the city (transport was provided between sites but this was far from ideal). Although the scientific programme was of a very high standard, the Institute received a large number of complaints from members about the organisation of the meeting and the quality of the accommodation – student bedrooms with shared and sometimes semicommunal bathrooms and toilets. Members attending conferences had come to expect a more integrated meeting with comfortable and convenient rooms. In spite of the problems, feedback from members on the scientific and social programme was complimentary; nevertheless, it was clear that time had come for change.

***

After much discussion, and a report from the conference committee, Council decided to look for professional conference organisers to undertake all the administrative arrangements in the name of the Institute and to try to find a venue more suited to the needs of a prestigious conference. The only aspect of the organisation retained by the Institute was the design of the scientific programme. After discussions with four companies and reviewing a number of possible venues, Reed Exhibitions was selected as conference organiser and the Birmingham International Conference Centre was selected as the most suitable venue.

During 1992 the Institute developed the Company Membership scheme and a Company Members Liaison Group comprising industry representatives and Institute officers was formed. This was perhaps fortuitous as it provided a forum for the discussion of the problems experienced during the Liverpool Triennial. By keeping potential exhibitors informed of developments and taking heed of their views, when the decision to completely revamp the Conference was taken (it was relaunched as the Biomedical Science Congress in 1995) it had the support and the assistance of the Company Members.

There can be no doubt that the smooth running of Congress owed, and continues to owe, a great deal to the considerable support from branch members in the Midlands who had gained experience from organising the 1989 Triennial in Warwick. Without their help in the background, packing Congress bags, manning the information desk and escorting speakers to and from the lecture theatres, things could have been much more difficult.

***

Notwithstanding the problems with the Triennial meeting held in Liverpool in 1992, overall the Conference meetings series was a resounding success. Over a period of 68 years the 22 conferences or weekend study courses did what they set out to do when the first was held in 1924 to great acclaim – to facilitate the formal and informal exchange of ideas and practices, help to develop contacts and improve the corporate identity of the Association and its members. There can be no doubt that the objectives were not only achieved but surpassed. If the number of participants can be taken as an indicator of success then the rise from around 80 at the first meeting to a peak in attendance of over 2300 demonstrates that the meetings were very successful. They were organised by Institute members for the Institute and its members and the pathology community at large and they also reached out to educate and inform the general public.

Chapter 7

A Society on Which the Sun Never Set

Open any world atlas during the first half of the 20th century and one thing would be immediately apparent: much of the global land mass was coloured red. This hue denoted membership of the British Empire, which comprised Dominions, Colonies, Protectorates, Mandates and other territories ruled or administered by the United Kingdom. King George VI was the last English monarch to be styled Emperor, but his successor, Queen Elizabeth II, continues to head the Commonwealth of Nations that evolved subsequently, and on which the sun never sets.

Albert Norman and the other founding members were men of vision, but even they would have been surprised and pleased to see how the Association developed worldwide and how it became the inspiration for the formation of similar associations across the globe.

At the beginning of the 20th century the British Empire, as it was then – the Commonwealth as it is now – was described as an 'Empire on which the sun never set'. From the outset, the PBLAA had an international membership drawn from this Empire. As the Dominions and Colonies of the Empire became independent and self-governing, the Institute and its members, directly or indirectly, were able to assist in the formation and development of similar professional bodies in the countries of the Commonwealth. Additionally, being one of the earliest, if not the earliest, professional body for medical laboratory scientists (it is certainly the longest surviving body) its expertise proved invaluable to countries in other parts of the world including the European Union.

The initial proposal to form an association was circulated across the network of laboratory assistants known to be working in British university and research laboratories in 1911, but the news of the association spread rapidly outside the UK. Consequently, within the first year there were applications from three gentlemen working overseas: in Sudan, Ceylon and from a Mr T Whyte from Montreal, Canada. A motion to accept members from abroad, and to encourage them to form branches, was passed at the January 1913 meeting of the committee. The minutes for 1913 show that there were three members in Canada, three in Sudan and one in New Zealand.

How these men came to learn about the association is not known. Some assistants were employed by the Colonial Office, others by UK research laboratories. W J Muggleton, who worked for the London School of Tropical Medicine, wrote of his experiences as a laboratory assistant in the Crown Colony of Fiji, 14,000 miles from London, in Volume 1 of *The Laboratory Journal*. By 1916 there were members in British South Africa, Canada, India, New Zealand, Sudan and Uganda. As the number of overseas members increased it was agreed that it was a 'sound idea' to form a division to represent overseas members. The minutes from 1922 suggest that they were particularly concerned for the members in the Protectorates – a Protectorate, in the then British Empire, was a territory not formally annexed but in which, by treaty, grant or other lawful means, the Crown had power and jurisdiction – and in 1924 W J Muggleton was appointed as Overseas Corresponding Secretary. The overseas members were as enthusiastic as their UK-based colleagues – there is a report that it was "hoped to arrange with Mr Baily to arrange at Nairobi a few meetings of the Assistants in the Kenya Colony". Periodically, the expatriates came home on leave, some to study at the London School of Hygiene and Tropical Medicine. For others, the Association helped to arrange study facilities in appropriate laboratories.

An Overseas Committee, with Messrs Muggleton, Berry, Bromfield, Deacon and Signy as members, was established by the IMLT in 1944 and international standing of the IMLT is perhaps best demonstrated by the overseas section of the IMLT Annual Report for that year.

> The Governments of many of the Allied Nations have agreed that on repatriation they will look to the Institute for guidance in establishing organisations of a similar nature in their own countries.
>
> Contact has been made with the Registry of Medical Technicians of America, the Society of Laboratory Technicians of Australia, The Association of Scientific Workers of South Africa, and the Canadian Society of Medical Laboratory Technicians.
>
> The Senior Medical Officer of the European U.N.R.R.A [United Nations Relief and Rehabilitation Administration] has agreed to recruit laboratory technicians only through the Institute, as have the Council of Societies for Relief Abroad.
>
> The Colonial Office continues to notify the Institute of vacancies in the Colonies, and contact has been made with all Dominion Governments.
>
> The Council has consented to a proposal to hold the Institute in the Colonies or elsewhere where the demand exists, and for the establishment of branches in the Colonies and for the affiliation of other organisations to the Institute. The Council continues to investigate the matter on behalf of the Council *(sic)*.

***

The International standing of the Institute is further illustrated by events that took place in the early 1970s.

Following discussion between the Commonwealth Foundation (CF) – an intergovernmental body established by the Commonwealth Heads of Government in 1965 – and John Fawcett in 1972 it was agreed that the IMLS would investigate the development of the profession within the Commonwealth. The secretaries of appropriate societies and, where these did not exist, relevant interested local personnel were asked for information on the development of the profession within their countries. Not all countries replied and the details from each that did varied in detail. W J Fincham collated the responses and his analysis formed the substance of a report which was discussed at a conference, under the chairmanship of F J Baker, IMLS President, in January 1976. The IMLS was also represented by W J Fincham and J K Fawcett, and there were representatives for Australia, Sierra Leone, Guyana and Nigeria together with A G Beer from the World Health Organization (WHO) with knowledge of Sri Lanka and Bangladesh. It is interesting to note that all of the participants, with the exception of the Australian representative, were either Fellows or Associates of the Institute.

At the opening of the meeting, it was explained that by working within the framework of the Commonwealth cooperation it was hoped to identify areas of technology where help might be needed and a grant of £10,000 be allocated to help pursue this aim.

Following discussion of the report and visits to The University Hospital of Wales in Cardiff, The London Hospital laboratories and Paddington College, various recommendations were made. These were published by the CF under the title *Problems Facing the Medical Laboratory Profession within the Commonwealth* and this formed the basis for further development.

Among the proposals were regular zonal meetings and the formation of a secretariat to coordinate these developments, and the CF agreed to provide funds for the IMLS to take on this role.

***

The first overseas branch to be formed was in Australia. Soon after the formation of the PBLAA, laboratory assistants in Sydney, Australia, learnt about the Association, at a meeting of 20 assistants on 26 June 1913 they decided to form a branch of the PBLAA and sent the following letter to Albert Norman.

Dear Sir

It was with great pleasure that the Laboratory Assistants of Sydney heard of the formation of your Association.

We are of the opinion that a very strong branch could be formed in Australia, and an endeavour is being made to organise the other States.

If your Association would supply us with a number of copies of the rules and Journal, it would help us greatly in our organising, as the Journal illustrates the aims and objects of the Association better than can be done by letter.

A provisional committee has been formed, and the Pathological Society of New South Wales is being asked for its support.

We shall be pleased to receive any further information that you may deem it advisable to forward

With hearty good wishes for the success of the Association.

S Birrell

Hon. Sec., *pro tem.*

A provisional committee was formed, which, due to an outbreak of smallpox in Sydney, was unable to meet until 2 June 1914. At a general meeting on 9 June it was resolved that the branch be formed as from 1 July 1914. The report in the September edition of *The Laboratory Journal* shows there were 23 members and four juniors, and efforts were being made to enrol members in six other cities. By 1916, membership had risen to 35, including members in Melbourne.

As the members of the Australian branch worked in the various departments that supported the Medicine and Veterinary faculties, the PBLAA certificate examinations were not suitable for them. As a result, it was decided to withdraw from the PBLAA and form an association more suited to Australian conditions. This became the Medical Sciences Laboratory Assistants Association (MSLAA), later to become the Society of Laboratory Technicians and then The Australian Institute of Medical Scientists. The new body recognised the value of *The Laboratory Journal* and continued to purchase copies for its members. It was also suggested that MSLAA members, when visiting Britain, should be honorary members of PBLAA, and vice versa. A further manifestation of this agreement appeared in 2005 when it was agreed that Membership of the Australian Institute of Medical Scientists was equivalent to Fellowship of the Institute.

***

The Nigerian branch was formed in 1960 but in the early 1970s the Institute of Medical Laboratory Technology Nigeria emerged, which developed its own examinations and qualification system. It retains close links with the IBMS and many Nigerians hold dual membership. The 1972 report by the CF indicated that the development of the profession in Nigeria was the most advanced in Africa at that time.

The formation of a branch of the IMLT in Hong Kong was approved by Council in 1975 and despite major political changes it remains an active branch within the Institute. Two new overseas branches were formed in 1991, in Cyprus in April and Gibraltar in May.

***

In the early 1920s the formation of an Association of Bacteriologists was proposed in New Zealand by Tom Ross from Christchurch and Andrew Logan from Dunedin. The PBLAA records for 1913 show that there was one member from New Zealand and that a T Ross joined in the same year as an overseas member. There are no surviving records of formal contact between the PBLAA and the New Zealand Association, but it is most likely that Tom Ross and T Ross are one and the same person and that his inspiration probably came from the UK.

It is interesting to note that the timing of the proposal coincides with the introduction of the certification scheme in the UK, and that this was one of the major reasons for the formation of an independent body in Australia. The idea gained little support from senior pathologists, but in 1923 a number of staff from Wellington Hospital, supported by the pathologist, Dr Hector, met to discuss the proposal. This led to the drawing up and printing of the *Constitution and Rules of the Bacteriological and Pathological Association of New Zealand (1925)*. Probably because of the Depression, the Association did not take off and in 1937 a further attempt was made. Again nothing happened and the outbreak of war in 1939 hampered any development. In 1945, Laurie Buxton, who had been involved in the first meeting in 1923, convened a meeting which led to the formation of The New Zealand Association of Bacteriologists in 1946. In 1990, this became the New Zealand Institute of Medical Laboratory Science.

***

Originally, PBLAA members in Ireland were members of the Belfast branch, which, together with Edinburgh and Glasgow formed Division D. When the IMLT adopted a region and branch structure in 1947 an Irish region was established. The regional centre was in Belfast, with George McKee as convener and regional representative. By that time there were branches in both Belfast and Dublin, and much later branches were established in Limerick and Cork. When the Republic of Ireland was established, links with the IMLT, and its examinations system, were retained. The practical Intermediate examinations alternated, spring and autumn, between Belfast and Dublin, with senior members of the profession from both centres acting as examiners.

When the Intermediate and Final examinations were replaced in the UK by the ONC/OND and HNC/HND qualifications, the Department of Education in the Republic of Ireland, with help from the IMLT, set up comparable courses in 1968. These allowed successful candidates to continue to qualify for Membership and Associateship of the Institute.

Eventually, the decision was made to create Ireland's own professional body and in 1974 the Academy of Medical Laboratory Science was established. Many Irish members retained their association with the Institute and there are still branches in Dublin and Limerick with a combined membership in 2010 of around 156.

The collaboration between the two bodies was further strengthened in 1995 when the Academy's scientific journal *The Journal of Biomedical*

Sciences was incorporated into the *British Journal of Biomedical Science*.

***

As has been seen, there was educational activity in Kenya in the early years of the PBLAA and there were individuals working in East Africa. In the late 1930s there was an attempt to form an East Africa branch of the PBLAA. Sydney Laws, who was working in Uganda, proposed its formation and went as far as to designate himself as 'Corresponding Member for East Africa to the PBLAA' and also 'Potential Secretary, East Africa Branch PBLAA' . However, this was without the approval of the Association and he was admonished for his presumption. The branch was never established and whether or not this was because of the differences with Sydney Laws, the changes following the Second World War or the formation of the IMLT is not clear.

Although formal branches were not established, reports in *The Gazette* in 1955 indicate that there were active groups of members both in Kenya and in Salisbury, Southern Rhodesia. From these reports it is evident that the IMLT examinations were important for those working in East Africa, as the conditions of service for East Africa specified that IMLT qualifications were required in order to pass promotion bars in the salary scales.

Intermediate examinations were conducted in the various countries of the area. In the 1960s and 1970s many men and women came to the UK, on scholarships, to train and to sit the examinations for Associateship and Fellowship. It was these men and women who, on return to their own countries, established education systems within their own countries. Between 1967 and 1977 the Inter-University Council of East Africa took over the training, examination and award of certificate and diploma qualifications to successful students from the IMLT in the UK. With the break up of the East African Community in 1977, individual countries took over their role. Both Kenya and Uganda have professional bodies that are members of the International Federation of Biomedical Laboratory Science (IFBLS).

***

The International Association of Medical Laboratory Technologists (IAMLT) was founded in 1954. Although the brainchild of the Swiss, who held the secretariat from 1954 to 1973, the Institute, through the size of its membership and therefore its financial contribution, had an important influence on its development. The meeting to draft a constitution for the IAMLT was held at the 1955 Triennial Conference and when its first Council was elected, in 1958, R J Broomfield, the then IMLT Chairman, became the first President, a position he held until 1961.

The Institute continued to play a dominant role in the Association. When, in 1977, the Executive Director resigned, Guy Pascoe agreed to take on the secretarial duties in addition to his Presidential duties. He continued to serve as the Executive Director until 1980, although his term as President ended in 1978. Besides holding the vital post of President and Executive Director, he was also recording secretary and Editor of *Medical Technology International* during his term of office as a council member. The Presidency was also held by Dennis Slade and Graham Smart, the latter for two terms; Dennis was also Editor of *Medical Technology International* in 1985/86 and 1989/90.

Despite this involvement, in 1995 the then President, David Browning, proposed that the Institute should resign from the IAMLT. He felt that it had become too introspective and proposed an alternative based on a WHO model. The proposal was not without its opponents, but Council supported the President and the Institute left the IAMLT in 1995.

In 2010 the IBMS rejoined what had become the IFBLS. It took the view that as the IFBLS had a growing record of political influence, worked closely with WHO and was actively involved with ISO standards, it was important that the Institute was involved with and contributed to these activities.

***

Following the United Kingdom's decision to join the European Community, the Institute took the lead in the formation of the Standing Representative Committee (SRC) for Medical Laboratory Technology at a meeting hosted by the IMLT in 1973. The role of the SRC was to act in a consultative capacity, providing advice to the European Commission on matters of importance to the profession. The IMLT had four representatives on the original body: Frank

Baker, who became the first chairman, John Fawcett, the first secretary, Tom Lansley and Guy Pascoe.

The Institute continued to provide both the Chairman and Secretary until it amalgamated with the IAMLT's European group to form the European Association for Professions in Biomedical Science (EPBS). The aims of this new body were to raise the profile of the professional and to develop professional standards. Martin Nicholson was elected the first EPBS President in its inaugural year, a position he held until 2004. During his tenure he was an energetic advocate of involving prospective biomedical scientists in developing the future shape of the profession. To this end, he established a students' forum within the EPBS that is tasked with developing policy ideas which continue to be presented for inclusion by the EPBS general assembly of delegates in EPBS policy.

Martin began the process of establishing common agreement on training and education standards (albeit an aspiration only for some nations in Europe). The EPBS has since agreed that education should be to Cycle One of the Bologna Process and include a period of clinical training in placement and be to the equivalent of 240 European Credit Accumulation and Transfer System (CATS) points. The pursuit of a European register of biomedical scientists was an idea that commenced during Martin's presidency, but is only now being discussed more actively. Martin sought to have the EPBS set up as a credible legal entity and in 2006 it became registered as such in Belgium. In 2005 the IBMS withdrew from membership of EPBS but rejoined in 2008.

In 1994 the IBMS joined the European Confederation of Laboratory Medicine (now European Laboratory Medicine) and the Institute was represented by Martin Nicholson, who was also Treasurer from 1998 to 2004, when IBMS membership ceased.

In response to the growing number of European initiatives, in 1992 a European Affairs Committee of Council was established. This allowed it to deal in a more cohesive manner with the increasing influence of Europe. Some initiatives were aimed at professional and educational matters but others dealt with safety, standardisation of laboratory materials and reagents, and, in more recent times, the cross-recognition of qualifications within the

European Union, and with CE marking.

When the IBMS resigned its membership of the IAMLT it could no longer be a member of the European group of the IAMLT, the European Confederation of Medical Laboratory Technologists Associations (ECMLTA). However, it continued to be a member of the SRC and at this time was represented by Martin Nicholson. At this time the SRC and ECMLTA were holding joint meetings and Martin was instrumental in persuading the two to reorganise into a stand-alone entity for Europe. As testament to these efforts, the EPBS was formed in 1999 as the single representative body.

***

The devolution of responsibility for healthcare to the parliaments of Northern Ireland, Scotland and Wales presented a new challenge to the IBMS. Although healthcare had, to a greater or lesser extent, been within the purview of the Secretaries of State for Scotland, Wales and Northern Ireland, matters concerning the profession were handled more or less consistently across the UK. With the transfer of responsibility, different approaches developed in the devolved administrations, requiring the Institute to develop new arrangements for dealing with these new bodies. Notwithstanding these differences, there is no doubt that the vast majority of the membership will continue to develop their practice to ensure high-quality care, and, irrespective of the fact that the model of delivery may be different within the home countries of the UK, the fundamental biomedical science practice will remain of a similar high quality.

The interests of biomedical scientists in Northern Ireland are looked after by the Northern Ireland branch which is also responsible for political lobbying in the Northern Ireland Assembly.

In Scotland a devolved Scottish committee of the IBMS was initiated after the new parliament for Scotland was created in May 1999. It is the recognised region of the IBMS and the main route between the Scottish branches and Council.

A distinct role for IBMS in Scotland is as the professional conduit between the Scottish Government and the body of biomedical scientists practising in Scotland. Representatives from the biomedical scientist community in Scotland sat on many influential committees to inform the development of health policy and the biomedical science role in informing that policy.

A significant element of change from a biomedical science perspective was the role of IBMS in Scotland in the creation and working of the Biomedical Science Modernisation Board. This resulted in the development of a coherent national plan designed to address recruitment and retention issues. This involved a national programme for integrated degrees and, through NHS Education Scotland, funding for placement officers. Following development of the Healthcare Science Strategy for Scotland, launched in 2007, the IBMS worked closely with the Scottish Government to ensure developments in Scotland aligned with the UK *Modernising Scientific Careers* programme.

Devolution had little impact on the function of the IBMS in Wales, which had always had a scientific advisory structure. Through discipline-specific advisory groups, this advised the laboratory services committee which in turn advised the Welsh Scientific Advisory Committee, the chair of which advised the Minister. This arrangement continued after devolution. Although the Institute was not formally represented on these groups, membership was drawn from senior laboratory staff and thus senior members of the Institute.

Chapter 8

The PBLAA, the Outbreak
of the Second World War,
and the Chidwick Letters

*In 1938, British Prime Minister Neville Chamberlain referred to
Czechoslovakia as a "country far away" and a "people of which we know
nothing". In the seven decades since he alighted an airplane with a letter in
hand, in the wake of technological advances in aviation and communication
which mean that travel to the Antipodes takes no more than 24 hours, and
electronic communication is almost instantaneous, such sentiments are
seriously outdated and yet sadly prescient.*

On the announcement of war in September 1939, there were immediate limitations on travel and the availability of members of the PBLAA Council. It was quickly agreed to establish a War Emergency Committee to take over the functions of Council. A meeting was convened by Mr C E Layng, Vice President, on Sunday 17 September 1939, at 36 Kingshill Avenue, Kenton, Middlesex – the home of Mr W J Muggleton.

Layng chaired the meeting and it was attended by S J Denyer (Secretary), F R Croxon (Treasurer), Albert Norman (Editor, *The Laboratory Journal*), F R Chopping (Examining Council), R J Bromfield (Editor, *Monthly Bulletin*), W J Muggleton (Prize Fund Committee) and B E Gilbey (Division A [London] representative). The chairman explained the purpose of the meeting and it was agreed to ask Council to vest its powers in the War Emergency Committee to maintain the interests of the PBLAA and its members. The new committee would consist of the above named officers, with authority to co-opt other members of the Council, with a proviso that four members were required to form a quorum.

W J Muggleton agreed to become Honorary Secretary of the new committee and he was immediately tasked with contacting other Council members not present in order to seek their approval for the transfer of authority. The members of the War Emergency Committee all lived in the London area, with the exception of Sidney Denyer, who lived in Yorkshire, as it was thought it was easier for them to meet, hence the appointment of Muggleton as the new secretary.

The new War Emergency Committee's first action was to cancel the Part I examinations planned for November 1939 and consider holding them the following year. There was, however, strong support for maintaining publication of *The Laboratory Journal* and the *Monthly Bulletin* and encouragement for continuing divisional activities around the country. The committee also considered the safeguarding of PBLAA records and agreed that satisfactory arrangements were in place. Proof of their diligence in this respect is the continuing existence of all PBLAA archives.

Ongoing plans to make the PBLAA a company were considered and Mr Denyer was instructed to seek clarification with the professional body's legal advisor, Mr Chidwick, to see if it was possible to continue their application, but to defer taking over the actual role of a company. It was later decided to gain all possible information required to proceed towards the registration of a company with the minimum of delay, taking fresh legal advice if required.

***

It is of interest that the PBLAA secretariat was consulted regularly on salary levels for particular experienced staff and the War Department had requested advice on a suitable salary for laboratory assistants with specialist experience who were deployed in the Armed Services. The level quoted was £5 per week, equivalent to the pay of an Army Sergeant. Such was the frequency of requests for similar information that an article entitled 'The War and the Laboratory Technician' was published in the *Monthly Bulletin* in 1940.

At a meeting of the War Emergency Committee, on 28 April 1940, it was announced that a memorandum of the proposed company formation had been lodged with the Board of Trade, its assets being stated as £2980 9s 8d (£2980 46p) in the application.

It was reported at the next meeting, on 1 September 1940, that the Board of Trade had objected to the inclusion of the employment bureau function of the proposed company, as detailed in the memorandum. It was agreed to accept this deletion, in order to forward the application process.

The committee met again on 21 September 1940 to consider the minutes of the last Annual General Meeting of the PBLAA, which took place on 18 February 1939. The secretary announced that he was unable to provide copies of the Annual Report, as they had been sent to a stenographer for copying "but were now at the bottom of a heap of rubble, all that remains of her premises after being bombed by German airmen". At this meeting, it was also decided that £400, previously to be placed on investment, be lent to H M Government, free of interest. A further £1000 of PBLAA funds was used to purchase 3% Defence Bonds (ie loaning the money to the Government). Thus, it cannot be said that the PBLAA did not do its duty to the country in time of need.

Owing to the increasing pressure on finances, partly due to a fall in subscriptions and advertising revenues, it was decided to suspend publication of *The Laboratory Journal* for the duration of the War, but to continue producing the *Monthly Bulletin*.

***

At the War Emergency Committee meeting on 2 February 1941, two issues occupied the minds of the Committee, and both seem quite extraordinary by modern standards. It was agreed by the committee that "Technicians of other than British birth be not accepted for membership of this Association". This decision was taken in view of the fact that refugees from Europe then domiciled in the country would attempt or had already attempted to join the Association.

The second matter concerned the issue of women taking up posts to replace technicians who had been conscripted was discussed and left on the table; translated, this meant that a decision could not be agreed. In the situation, it was decided this issue would be taken up with the President for further advice.

Such were the views of that day and age!

***

Members of the PBLAA, in particular those already holding the qualifying Certificate, were questioning their lack of recognition and subsequent suppressed remuneration. There were calls for the state registration of 'medical laboratory technicians' as they were now called and other members believed that only the awarding of a Royal Charter would meet their requirements.

In early 1936, following nearly four years of negotiations, the Board of Trade approved the formation of the Board of Registration of Medical Auxiliaries; this enabled a national register of health practitioners to be established. The bodies initially included the Society of Apothecaries, the British Medical Association, the Chartered Society of Massage and Medical Gymnasts, and the Society of Radiographers. The purpose of the register was intended to list bona-fide qualified practitioners in their respective professions for referrals from medical doctors. The Articles of Association of the new

Board fell short of preventing non-registrants from practising, unlike the register of dentists, just created, which did achieve this. Some believed that the PBLAA should seek registration with the new Medical Auxiliaries Board, which was thought possibly to be a better option than 'state registration'.

One member was particularly active in seeking the Council of the PBLAA to pursue a pathway toward achieving inclusion on such a register. In 1936, Sidney Laws, while on leave in Newcastle from his post in Uganda, wrote to Sidney Denyer, the PBLAA General Secretary, to commend efforts towards applying for a Royal Charter or becoming recognised through some form of state registration.

His letters are reproduced below.

Newcastle upon Tyne
8 July 1936

Dear Denyer,

Many thanks for your note and good wishes. I am looking forward to the Conference and meeting with all my old friends again.

I have asked the Secretary to send to you a copy of the Memorandum and Articles of Association and Byelaws of the Board of Registration of Medical Auxiliaries, which has just been incorporated, and trust this may be of great interest to you if you have not already heard of it. Maybe the Council could consider this before the Conference meets in August and some statement made for the information of members.

I am going to ask if anything definite has been done about the Royal Charter and whether this would be advisable considering the cost, and the advantages to be gained, and whether qualified legal advice has been sought on a question affecting the future of the Association. I am making a few enquiries and would like to know whether you would like me to go on with it or not! I would like to know for my own information, but if you would not like it brought up for discussion just let me know.

I am hoping that something will be done soon, as I am sure you are, as I know how keen you have been about the whole point.

I have asked for a copy of the Memorandum to be sent to Norman who I know will be interested if he has not already seen it.

In the meantime, my apologies for troubling you

With kind regards
Yours very sincerely
S.G.Laws

Meanwhile, Laws had written to the Registrar of the Board of Medical Auxiliaries, which resulted in him suggesting a meeting between himself and Sidney Denyer. Laws' second letter to Sidney Denyer, just a few days later, is most significant in his suggestion to seek incorporation under the Companies Act.

Newcastle upon Tyne
10 July 1936

Dear Denyer,
    Further to my letter of a few days ago.
For some time I have been thinking over the suggestion that the Association should make application for a Royal Charter with power to grant a diploma. Since I arrived home I have made a few enquiries as to the method of application, costs, advantages etc., but have found it very difficult, as no one seems to know how to go about it. I have been informed that the services of a Parliamentary Agent would be necessary and considerable influential and financial backing would have to be forthcoming to meet with success, as the application has to go before the Privy Council. I have wondered if we would have the support of the Medical and Veterinary bodies? I am rather doubtful. I have also been told that a recent application by the Institute of Municipal and County Engineers has been turned down. Probably you have more information at your disposal as to the chance of success and the costs entailed.
    May I suggest to you another method of approach?
I think that the same advantages could be gained by incorporation under the Companies Act as a Company limited by guarantee. This would not be such an expensive method, would give the same advantages as a Royal Charter and I believe some additional ones.
    In my searches I came across the new body started by the B.M.A and other auxiliary bodies, which might be helpful to the Association. When I asked the Secretary to send you particulars, I also asked him about the method of applying for a Royal Charter and the probable cost, also if registration under the Companies Act would give the same advantages.

As the first General Meeting has also been held, I asked for a copy of the proceedings as this would tell more of the functions of the Board and the scope of the Register. I have had a reply and enclose it with this letter. If you think it worthwhile and can spare the time, probably you will look him up as he suggests.

In the meantime I am waiting for a reply to some legal queries and will probably get more precise information upon Parliamentary Agents, costs, method of application for Royal Charter, Companies Act etc., and I will let you have all the information as soon as possible. I have a copy of the Companies Act, 1929, and I will let you have this later, if of any use to you.

Anything else that I could do I would be only too pleased if this would help along the objects you have in mind.

With sincere regards

Yours

S G Laws

***

The 5th Triennial Conference of the PBLAA took place in Edinburgh in August 1936 and proved to be a pivotal event in the development of the Association. Sidney Laws spoke at length on his research concerning options for the Association to take on a formal status. His ideas received wide support, in particular that of incorporation of the Association into a company limited by guarantee under the Companies Act.

The matter was considered by Council and in September 1937 the General Secretary, Sidney Denyer, was instructed to seek learned opinion on the subject and £30 was agreed for this purpose. Denyer approached Mr Eric Chidwick FCIS, a chartered secretary, to examine the process (and costs) of forming the existing Association (PBLAA) into a company. Mr Chidwick's letter of response to Council is a seminal document in the establishment of the Institute.

49 Holders Hill Avenue
Hendon
NW4
September 1937

Gentlemen,

I have been requested by Mr S J Denyer your Secretary to explore the possibilities of registering the Association as a limited liability company under the Companies Act 1929.

It would appear that it would be advisable (if the project go forward) to register the word INSTITUTE, and which company would be limited by guarantee.

It should be explained that a company (amongst other methods) may be a company with a share capital made up of a given number of shares of a certain value. Supposing this certain value to be £1 then a Member holding 100 shares would pay £100 for those shares and his liability is limited to the said sum of £100. If the total share capital amounts to say £10,000, this sum is of course available for the purpose of the Company's trading.

In the case of the Association it is not proposed to adopt this method as no monies are required for purposes similar to those outlined above. The method suggested is to form a Company limited by guarantee, which means that Members are not called upon to subscribe Capital in pounds sterling but each Member will guarantee to subscribe to the funds of the Company (if required) up to a previously agreed figure.

For instance, a Member may guarantee up to say £10 and if the company were at any time to become insolvent, that Member must find £10 towards the deficiency but NO MORE. In order to Register a Company it is required to prepare certain documents the most important of which are known as the Memorandum and Articles of Association and these documents are in fact the Rules and Regulations which govern the Company.

The Memorandum of Association requires particular care in compilation because the Company takes its power to conduct any business from this document, and any power not given in this document can never be acquired, in other words the company cannot legally do anything for which power is not given in the Memorandum of Association, full provision should therefore be given for anything which IS, or MAY at any time, be required. The Articles of Association are the ordinary Rules upon which the Company bases its everyday life, and this document can be altered to suit circumstances, by a Resolution of the Company at a Meeting of its Members but of course the Articles are always subject to the Memorandum.

The advantages of forming the Association into such a Company is that instead of as at present relying upon the enthusiasm of certain individuals, the Association would become a body corporate whose existence would be governed by its whole membership, each member taking an active part in the government of the Company.

It should be explained that a Company unlike an individual, never dies, in other words it is an artificial, but quite legal, personality which is created by the operation of the law in the form of the Companies Act 1929.

It would be necessary to draft these Memorandum and Articles of Association for the consideration of the Council, should they decide to form a Company.

I have had the opportunity of perusing your present Rules and literature and have given the matter my serious consideration. I am of opinion that a suitable company could be formed, should you so decide, and would be willing to have the aforementioned documents ready for your consideration when you next meet, upon receiving instructions from your Mr Denyer.

Eric C Chidwick FCIS

Denyer then sent copies of this letter to Council members with a questionnaire, which sought to identify opinion on the key points raised in the 'Chidwick Letter'.

The variation of responses and considerable correspondence which this generated must have been an additional burden for Denyer, who, in addition to his increasing secretarial duties for the PBLAA, also had a full-time post in the laboratory, where he earned his living.

The scope of opinion expressed ranged from outright rejection by the Division B representatives from Birmingham and Cardiff, through cautious progress to complete acceptance towards seeking incorporation as a company as described.

Undaunted, Denyer asked Chidwick to respond to the points of most concern identified by members to his original letter. Chidwick composed a second letter with answers and explanations.

49 Holders Hill Avenue
Hendon
NW4
October 1937

Gentlemen,

I understand from Mr S J Denyer that the original Memorandum which I prepared for him has been circularised to various Members of your Council and that a representative proportion of Council Members have replied asking a number of questions on the matter under consideration.

I have endeavoured to set out these questions and as far as possible to answer each query, as follows:

1.   Should we require to have a Registered Office, and would it be 'open' to members?
Answer – Yes, a Registered Office is required, although there is no reason that this should be situate other than at the residence of the Secretary.

2.   Should we require the services of a qualified man as Secretary to the Institute?
Answer – No, your Secretary could still do all that is required.

3.   To what extent would the annual expenditure increase?
Answer – The annual expenditure need not increase in any way.

4.   Would it be necessary to hold an ANNUAL General Meeting of Members?
Answer – Yes, this is required under the Companies Act, 1929.

5.   Surely we would require the services of a Solicitor to deal with the legal side of the registration?
Answer – No, that is quite unnecessary.

6.   What name is it proposed to Register?
Answer – This is entirely a matter for the Council but the selected name must be approved by the Registrar of Companies.

7.   What would be the cost of this very complicated process?
Answer – I estimate the total cost to be not more than £120, most of which will be expended on Stamp Duties, Registration fees, and printing and stationery.

8.   It is unreasonable to expect us to consider the Memorandum and Articles

of Association at a Council Meeting. Could we not have draft copies in advance? Answer – Yes, copies would be circulated to be in your hands for at least 3 weeks before the Council Meeting.

A number of Members think that I should not be asked to attend the Council Meeting, and I am of course quite willing to abide by your wishes in that matter.

I should like to mention that if you decide to have a draft of the proposed Memorandum and Articles submitted to you at your Meeting, and if you then decide to drop the matter, your only expense will be for typing the documents sent to you. No other expenses will have been incurred.

Members may like to know that my association with Mr Denyer in this matter is not for reasons of financial gain to myself, and I have informed your Secretary that my fee for the work you require executed will be 20 guineas, or, if you are unable to afford this fee, I shall be glad to give of my services entirely free of cost, as a mark of my personal regard for Mr Denyer.

Eric C Chidwick FCIS

***

The next stage of the process was the presentation of a Draft Memorandum and Articles of Association for the establishment of a Company or Institute, to the PBLAA Council on 12 February 1938. After debate, Council rejected the Draft but agreed that a nominated subcommittee comprising Frederick Chopping, Sidney Denyer, Bernard Gilbey, Charles Layng and Albert Norman should revise and redraft the document in a form to put to the PBLAA membership for approval.

After a year, and 18 meetings, the subcommittee finally produced a document which they considered would incorporate the founding values of the PBLAA while bringing the requirements to meet with Company law. At its first meeting in 1939, Council debated the new Draft and agreed the revision, with the aim to seek incorporation as a company with the registered title 'Institute of Medical Laboratory Technology'.

The proposal was put to the membership with a postcard response vote. The result was an overwhelming vote in favour to proceed: For 622, Against 47, Spoilt 5.

The timing of progress of this critical development of the old PBLAA to the new status of Institute of Medical Laboratory Technology (IMLT) could not have been more difficult. This had taken place against a background of rising military threats and invasions in Europe, eventually resulting in Britain's involvement in the Second World War.

In consideration of the devastating consequences of the early months of conflict in London and other major cities, it is remarkable that the bureaucratic passage involved in this transition made any progress. Eventually, in January 1942, a response was received from the Board of Trade that, subject to the withdrawal of a clause in the Memorandum of Association, the proposed Institute would act as an employment exchange, and the transformation of the PBLAA to IMLT could now be effected.

A public notice was placed in the *Daily Telegraph* and, subject to no objections being raised, the Board of Trade would issue a licence, registering the Institute of Medical Laboratory Technology as a limited liability company. This was received on 22 June 1942 and Council formally took over the assets, undertakings and functions of the PBLAA.

A meeting took place on 2 January 1943 of the Executive Council of the PBLAA and the Board of Directors of the IMLT, which formally marked the completion of the inception of the IMLT.

The Institute of Medical Laboratory Technology became a 'fully legal' body on the issue of the Certificate of Incorporation (No. 377288), which was issued and dated the 17th day of November 1942.

The amount of work involved during the six years leading up to the formation of the IMLT is difficult to assess accurately, but it certainly must have involved thousands of hours of letter-writing, research and countless meetings. All of this was done by those PBLAA Council members and a few others, in particular Sidney Laws. The most remarkable aspect is that they were also employed in laboratories across the country. Some, like Frederick Chopping, carried on working on the Council of the PBLAA for some time after his retirement from full-time employment.

The strain of the work involved is evident in some of the correspondence from members to Sidney Denyer, the General Secretary. Many sent their good wishes for his health, and commented on the amount of work that he was doing on behalf of the PBLAA.

It is therefore of no surprise that there were early discussions concerning the creation of a full-time General Secretary, as a further consequence of the siting of a Registered Office as part of the Memorandum of Association of the new Institute.

Profound gratitude must be accorded these people for their dedication and resilience in completing the creation of the Institute. This was done during a time of the worst disruption and threat to our very existence.

Chapter 9

Birth of the
Institute of Medical Laboratory Technology

Naturally, the history of the early 1940s is dominated by ongoing worldwide conflict; however, the 14th Academy Awards ceremony saw How Green Was My Valley *win Best Picture, the Oxford Committee of Famine Relief (OXFAM) founded, Walt Disney's animated film* Bambi *premiere in the UK, and a German rocket reach an altitude of over 80 miles above the earth, becoming the first man-made object, albeit briefly, to enter space.*

The Institute of Medical Laboratory Technology (IMLT) was officially born on 17 November 1942 on the issue of the Certificate of Incorporation by the Registrar of Companies. It had been a protracted gestation and a difficult birth, given the many issues that were debated in a period of wartime when the United Kingdom faced its gravest threat in history. The founding of the new Institute took place at a meeting held on Saturday 2 January 1943 at the London Nursing Home and Clinic at 149 Harley Street.

The meeting was initially convened as the 26th meeting of the Executive Council of the PBLAA and the first meeting of the Directors of the IMLT. Signatories to the Memorandum were present (excepting Andrew, Chopping, Hobson and Jelks). Also present were Hodgson, Dodds, Bush-Taylor, Chidwick (by invitation) and Deacon serving the interests of overseas members.

At the termination of the PBLAA business it was resolved at 6.58 pm that the PBLAA be dissolved and its assets and liabilities handed over to the IMLT, a resolution that was carried unanimously.

Sidney Denyer, long-time secretary of the PBLAA and whose tireless work was instrumental in achieving the creation of the Institute, was asked to open the meeting. In his introductory remarks he stated that it was the proudest day of his life. Denyer nominated Charles Layng as the first Chairman of the Institute, which was carried unanimously.

To enable the meeting to proceed to Election of Council, the election of Fellows was considered. Gilbey tendered his resignation under Article 20a, as not being eligible for Fellowship.

It was then resolved:

1   Applications for Fellowship be accepted from Bush-Taylor, Dodds and Hodgson, subject to the official forms being used, when available, also that the signatories to the Memorandum and Articles be accepted on the same conditions.

2   That the 15 nominations for Fellowship of the Company be accepted.

3   That Mr Gilbey be accepted as the first Associate.

4   Subject to the deletion of the names of Andrew, Gilbey and Jelks, the signatories to the Memorandum and Articles be elected the first Council, with the addition of Bush-Taylor, Dodds and Hodgson.

No. 377268.

Certificate of Incorporation

———

I HEREBY CERTIFY that INSTITUTE OF MEDICAL LABORATORY TECHNOLOGY (the word "Limited" being omitted by Licence of the Board of Trade) is this day incorporated under the Companies Act, 1929, and that the Company is Limited.

Given under my hand at Llandudno this Seventeenth day of November One thousand Nine Hundred and Forty-Two.

P. MARTIN,
Registrar of Companies.

The first Council of the Institute consisted of Messrs Norman, Chopping, Layng, Bromfield, Armstrong, Harper, Harvey, Male, Hobson, Bush-Taylor, Dodds, Herrick, Hodgson and Denyer – a total of 14 members. The officers elected to server were Professor J H Dible (President), A Norman (Vice Chairman), R Hodgson (Treasurer) and S J Denyer (Secretary).

***

The first meeting of the Council of the IMLT was held on 6 March 1943 at the Royal Hotel, Woburn Place, London. The President, Professor J H Dible, was in the Chair and those recorded as present were C E Layng, A Norman, R Hodgson, G Harper, G R Armstrong, T C Dodds, J L Herrick, C H B Taylor, H W Harvey, A Male, R J Bromfield, H Hobson and S J Denyer.

The minutes of this meeting reveal that there was a backlog of issues arising from the changeover from the PBLAA to the IMLT. There were a considerable number of PBLAA members serving in H M Forces throughout the world who had been unable to maintain their subscriptions. It was agreed that they should be admitted as Institute members once they resumed their subscriptions, waiving any amount outstanding since the outbreak of war in 1939.

The continuation of prize funds, such as the Sims Woodhead and Sidney Mann awards, established by the PBLAA, needed to be addressed due to the change of status, and the monies in the respective funds and, most significantly, the organisation of examinations needed urgent attention. A lot of work was required, much of it administrative, which fell upon the Secretary, Sidney Denyer. The first year of the new Institute was both eventful and turbulent. During 1943, the election to Council of Mr Richard Lavington (London) and Mr William Valentine (Exeter) would become probably the most significant decisions in developing the Institute during its early years. Both would go on to become the driving forces of the Institute for many years.

Sadly, the early death of Charles Layng, aged only 51, on 25 October just two days after chairing his last Council meeting, denied the Institute of a long-standing officer. He had served the PBLAA since 1922, becoming a Vice-President and Chairman of the Council and the first Chairman of the Institute.

George Harper took over as Chairman, temporarily, until a new election could take place.

On a positive note, and a sign of the developing organisation, approval was given to establish branches in Manchester, Leeds, Liverpool, Cardiff, Northern Ireland, Birmingham, Edinburgh, Glasgow, South Wales and London. A report to Council in May 1943 on Admissions to the Institute showed membership to be at 888 (Vice Presidents 3, Fellows 184, Associates 266, Members 346, Students 89).

Institute membership classes were based upon the design described by Sidney Laws at the PBLAA Conference at Edinburgh in 1936. He set out three classes, namely Student, Associate and Member. Students were persons not less than 16 years of age who had satisfied the Council as to a standard of general education, and who were in the course of training in an approved laboratory. They were required to present an annual report on the work performed during the year. Associates were persons who had at least three years' training in an approved laboratory since the date of registration as a Student and who had passed the Intermediate Examination. Members were persons who had been Associates for two years, who had at least five years' training in an approved laboratory since the date of registration as a Student, and who had passed the Final Examination.

The Institute (IMLT) decided to use the same classes but reversed the status of Members and Associates so that Associates were the 'qualified grade' and Members the 'unqualified grade'. This was contrary to most other professional organisations and caused a long-standing anomaly to overcome in comparative grading of members in status and salary terms.

The Institute also created the new class of Fellowship to be awarded to Associates who were successful in the Final Examination in a second subject. At the changeover from the PBLAA to the IMLT, Fellowship was also awarded to those who had previously been Registered Members of the PBLAA (having passed the Part II examination) and had been members of the PBLAA and of the Institute for a period of 10 years. A further group who had passed a major subject and held a special certificate in PBLAA examinations was granted Fellowship. From 1945, Fellowship could also be gained by thesis in exceptional cases.

Fellows were permitted to use the post-nominal letters FIMLT and Associates could use AIMLT, but members were not permitted to use MIMLT.

***

As a consequence of the many developments came an increasing administrative workload and at the Council meeting held on 23 October 1943, Sidney Denyer, Honorary Secretary, described the difficulties he was encountering and stated that it was no longer possible for an honorary officer to discharge the duties required. He urged Council to recruit a full-time official. Council agreed and advertisements for a General Secretary were placed in the *Daily Telegraph, Manchester Guardian, Yorkshire Post* and the Institute's *Monthly Bulletin*.

There were probably few members of the Council, especially the longer serving officers, who could have foreseen such a development before the first year of the new Institute had elapsed. Certainly, nobody would have foreseen the outcome of the impending appointment.

This decision demanded that premises be found to locate the appointed General Secretary and become the new Registered Office of the Institute. Two Council members (Bromfield and Lavington) were directed to find suitable accommodation.

Richard Lavington informed the Council meeting on 12 February 1944 that premises could be had at 15–16 Buckingham Street, Strand WC2, at a rental of £2 per week. The 'premises' consisted of a 14 x 10 foot room in a bomb-damaged building! Council agreed to accept this offer and arrange for the Registered Office to be transferred as convenient. It was also announced that 31 applications had been received for the post of General Secretary and, following shortlisting, four candidates "appeared before the Council". Mr James Maxwell Signy was selected and appointed for an initial period of six months at a salary of £400 per annum.

Signy, from London, had seen military service in the Army and Royal Air Force Volunteer Reserve and his background seemed appropriate, as he was a Fellow of the Royal Statistical Society and an Associate member of the

Institute of Industrial Administration and the Royal Institute of Public Health and Hygiene. Coincidentally, his brother, Dr A G Signy, was a well-known clinical pathologist; and would much later be one of the founders of The Royal College of Pathologists.

The year of 1944 was a landmark period in the development of the Institute, with the appointment of a salaried General Secretary in an independent Registered Office. Membership rose from 1052 to 1434, a 36% increase in the year, and the network of branches was extended to 17 when Council approved the formation of branches in the North East, Sheffield and Southampton. During 1944, 169 candidates entered Final Examinations in one of three subjects, Bacteriology, Pathology and Pathological Chemistry, and there were also 135 candidates for the Intermediate Examination.

***

The first meeting of the Joint Standing Committee of the Institute with representatives of the Pathological Society of Great Britain and Ireland and of the Association of Clinical Pathologists (ACP) took place on 21 September 1944. The meeting was chaired by Professor McIntosh and among the other medical representatives were Professor Dible (Institute President) and Dr Signy from the ACP. The Institute representatives were Albert Norman, Sidney Denyer, Richard Lavington and James Signy, the recently appointed General Secretary. He was also appointed Secretary to the Joint Standing Committee. Interestingly, soon after James Signy's appointment at the Institute, the Signy brothers would both become members of the same important committee, representing different organisations.

There had been cordial relations between the PBLAA and medical representatives for many years, with important decisions implemented only after joint agreement. The Institute was obviously keen to maintain this relationship, even though it was beginning to seek more independence in determining its strategies for the future, including its quest to secure a Royal Charter. There were other formal alliances to be created and, as a new organisation, it was important for the Institute to establish a position with key officials of government.

In this respect, a meeting between representatives of the Minister of Health and the Institute was held on 13 September 1944, when it was agreed that the Institute be recognised as a tutorial and qualifying body for medical laboratory technical personnel and that the Institute would be regarded as the appropriate body for consultation on matters of major importance in its area of activities. This is most significant as the Institute also received approval of its memorandum by health ministers, following the announcement of the government to establish a National Health Service.

The Institute also met with representatives of the (Armed) Services Pathological Departments under the chairmanship of Professor Dible, where agreement was reached whereby the training of medical laboratory technicians in the three Armed Services should conform to Institute standards, and the trainees would be encouraged to sit Institute examinations. It is clear that great efforts were made to establish and enhance the status of the Institute through the recognition of its education and qualification systems.

Two decisions, both indicating a positive attitude for the future, despite the continuation of war, were to recommence publication of *The Laboratory Journal*, which was suspended at the outbreak of war in 1939. The other was the announcement that an Institute library was to be established, following the donation of seven books.

All of these additional activities resulted in a request from the General Secretary for clerical support in the Registered Office. This was agreed, with a budget of £156 per annum, and subsequently the first appointee, a Miss Fairbairne, commenced work on a wage of £2 per week. It was also agreed to seek to extend the office premises occupied by the Institute, also with a budget of £156 per annum. This decision would be overtaken by the necessity to relocate the Registered Office several months later, during 1945.

***

During 1945 the United Kingdom saw the welcome end to nearly six years of hostilities across the world and the beginning of rebuilding normal civilian life.

The Institute witnessed a big increase in membership of more than 500 to a total of 1979 at the end of the year. Members were recorded as working in laboratories for government and municipal authorities as well as in the Armed Services, voluntary and independent hospitals, universities and research establishments.

The Registered Office was relocated to 12 Buckingham Street, Adelphi, London, following notice to quit on the return of the original tenants of the office at 15–16 Buckingham Street.

The Council of the Institute was faced with addressing an increasing number of queries concerning the re-integration of technicians returning from the Services to civilian posts. There was an admittance of its inadequacy in dealing with correspondence, especially concerning salary issues. This may seem inappropriate to the reader but in the 1940s the Institute was considered as a 'broker' in identifying appropriate salary levels for medical laboratory staff. There had been discussions between the Institute and the Association of Scientific Workers trades union, regarding salary issues. The Institute had clearly indicated that it did not seek a trades union role, but many members still believed and expected the Institute to perform this function, a situation that continued to cause dissatisfaction among the membership for many decades.

An indication of the direction of the Institute at this time can be seen in the format of the Council and its committee structure.

In 1946, five new branches were approved, which were Aberdeen, Colchester and Ipswich, Leicester, Preston and Reading. As a further result of increasing activity in the branches around the country, it was decided to create seven regions: London and South East, Midland, Western, Northern, Scotland, Ireland and Overseas.

With the exception of the Overseas region, each would send a representative to sit on Council. This was agreed at an Extraordinary General Meeting held on 1 June 1946 and resulted in changes to the Council membership, limiting nationally elected members to 15. The new regional members initially would be co-opted for one year until elections could take place, and all Council members would have equal voting rights. The regional appointments required that six existing members should retire, and Barker, Deacon, Lavington, Valentine, Wisdom and Jelks agreed to stand down.

The first regional Council members were approved at an Emergency Meeting of Council at The Kingsley Hotel in London on 3 November 1946, the appointees being R J Lavington (London and South East), G R Armstrong (Midland), G Harper (Western), S J Denyer (Northern), J L Herricks (Scotland) and G McKee (Ireland).

***

Despite the best-laid plans and an organisational structure in place, increasing problems became apparent in the running of the Institute administration. There were long delays in dealing with correspondence resulting in an increasing annoyance among members who had not received their membership diplomas. This reached such a pitch that the General Secretary, Mr Signy, had to publish an apology and an explanation for the delays, which appeared in *The Monthly Bulletin* in January 1946.

This, however, did not solve the problems and matters worsened until Council questioned Signy concerning his performance. In defence, he stated in a letter that "he had done his best" and that the facilities and staff in the Registered Office were insufficient to cope with the workload. This was probably true, given the sharp increase in membership issues as a result of the end of war, and the return of many members to civilian roles.

Signy sought a vote of confidence from Council, which was not forthcoming and subsequently tendered his resignation, which was accepted, with effect from 7 December 1946. This situation obviously threw the Institute into a crisis which was rescued through the appointment of two Council members. R J (Dickie) Lavington became Honorary Secretary with immediate effect on the resignation of Signy, and H A (Harry) Barker was appointed Honorary Treasurer, which was a new post. The General Purposes Committee was authorised by Council to manage the Institute office until the appointment of a new General Secretary.

The 'Signy Affair' was far from its conclusion, as on the compilation of the accounts for 1946 a "banking deficiency" involving a loss amounting to £1405 5s 3d (£1405 25p) was uncovered. This was equivalent to about a seventh of the Institute's total assets. Signy was sought to explain the loss, as

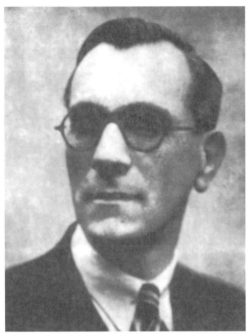

Sidney J Denyer

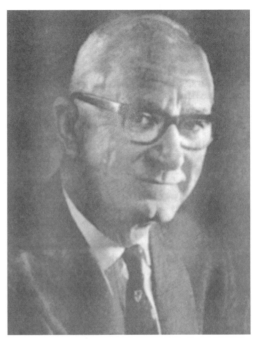

Richard J Lavington

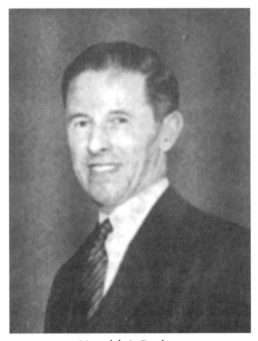

Harold A Barker

he had been responsible for financial affairs during his tenure as General Secretary. He eventually admitted responsibility for the losses and legal proceedings were initiated. The full amount was recovered during the ensuing months and no prosecution was instituted. Subsequent investigations by the Institute's auditors revealed that almost certainly there had been earlier misappropriations, which had remained undetected.

The whole affair ended with the Institute's finances intact and the appointment of devoted and loyal officers at the helm of the administration. They soon had to cope with yet another move for the Registered Office, when notice to vacate from 12 Buckingham Street was received. The new office was at 76 Brewer Street, close to Piccadilly, in Soho, gaining the benefit of additional accommodation by renting a large room divided into two on the fourth floor of the building.

The end of 1946 came with the news that the petition to the Privy Council for a Royal Charter had been rejected, completing a dark year in the early history of the Institute.

***

The development of the Institute is without doubt based on the people who were influential in its leadership and who carried out the essential business for the benefit of the membership. The appointment of Richard Lavington as Honorary Secretary and Harold Barker as Treasurer can be seen as the turning point to a successful period in the history of the Institute.

Both were long-standing members from the PBLAA, Richard Lavington was registered in 1920 and Barker in 1918; they had been members of the PBLAA Executive and brought a wealth of experience and stability to the Institute after the near disastrous period of Signy's term as General Secretary. In their respective ways, Lavington brought organisation and order to the Registered Office, and Barker took control of the finances through the careful scrutiny of spending and income during a time of increasing membership demands on the services of the Institute.

For a short time after his appointment, Lavington was given additional help in running the Registered Office through the appointment of an Assistant

Secretary, Mr S Hughes. Sadly, this arrangement was short-lived, as Hughes took up a post in Australia.

During 1947 the Council sought to re-establish the post of a full-time General Secretary and, following advertisements, five applicants emerged, among them Richard Lavington, who was appointed by unanimous approval of Council. He was probably the first laboratory man to make the changeover to becoming an administrator.

***

Richard Lavington, born in 1905, joined the PBLAA on commencement of work in London and maintained his membership through the transition to the IMLT and to his full-time administrative role.

Dickie Lavington, as he was known to his many colleagues, became a member of the PBLAA Executive Council in 1931, aged 26, and was instrumental in the establishment of the earliest examinations that would become the Intermediate. He represented the London branch and became the South East region Council member on the formation of the Institute in 1942. Following Signy's term as the first General Secretary, Dickie Lavington agreed to take on the role of Honorary Secretary of the Institute in December 1946. It soon became apparent that he would not be able to continue in his laboratory post and perform the role of Secretary in an effective manner. He commenced his new role in March 1948 and continued until his retirement in 1970, despite experiencing a heart attack. Dickie Lavington's contribution to the Institute was recognised through his awards of Life Membership in 1956, the Sims Woodhead Medal in 1969 and his election as a Vice President in 1970, shortly before his retirement.

He had an accomplished laboratory career with 28 years' experience in medical laboratories prior to his appointment as General Secretary. During this time he had contributed considerably to the PBLAA and the Institute and brought a sound knowledge of professional affairs to his new post. Dickie Lavington was a man of commanding appearance and, coupled with his administrative and financial skills, was perfectly suited to manage the rapidly expanding organisation that the Institute had become. He had considerable foresight and at a weekend conference at Blackpool in 1960 described the path that the Institute should take in reshaping the profession's education system that would gain national recognition while retaining the highest levels within Institute control.

Like all great men he had his idiosyncrasies, sometimes, in private, expressing a bizarre opinion, quite contrary to his position and normally astute manner. It was said that he saw no place for Whitley Council in determining salaries, believing that individuals in the caring professions should accept the conditions prevailing, however out of line, and not be involved in seeking betterment. A very strange stance for one charged with providing for the interests of a professional membership.

***

Harry Barker (1901–1957) began his career at the Middlesex Hospital in 1917 and developed a reputation as a skilled bacteriologist. He worked with luminaries such as Professor McIntosh and Sir Paul Fildes.

Harry Barker was appointed to the post of Treasurer of the Institute following the departure of J M Signy in December 1946, a role he held for more than 10 years until his death. This was a period of considerable expansion for the Institute and required very careful management of the finances due to increases in the cost of office accommodation, examinations and Institute publications. He proved well suited to the task as a man of firm beliefs. Such was his control of funds that he would not allow anything to be spent that might in any way be regarded as a benefit to individual members. As a result, members travelling to meetings in London were not even provided with a cup of tea!

Harry Barker had the misfortune to be profoundly deaf and as a result acquired a hearing aid device to allow him to follow the business at meetings. It was also a curious situation to new members of committees on which he sat that two seats would be left for him at the meeting table. One was for him and the other for his hearing aid machine which was of considerable dimensions and required constant adjustment of dials and switches. It was said anecdotally, perhaps unkindly, that he failed to hear financial requests of which he did not approve.

***

Harry Barker's period of office as Treasurer was a challenging one. The increase in Institute activities during the post-war years showed that concerns were mounting that the excess of income over expenditure (£1083) was reaching a critically low margin. There was an increase in costs associated with the Institute's publications, partly due to the decision to provide copies of *The Laboratory Journal* to Student members.

The relocation of the Registered Office to 9 Harley Street in November 1949 resulted in a three-fold increase in rent plus the cost of additional members of staff. A further concern for the Treasurer and Council was the diminishing returns from the Institute's investments, which were mainly in Government Stocks or Gilts. The income from membership fees had been affected by the disproportionately large number of Student members that had increased to 45% of membership by 1950. The reduced income from this group was considered the key factor in the overall financial position. It is also a recognition of the increased numbers of female students registering during the years 1948–50. However, it was thought that there would be a significant loss of those members after marriage.

Salary levels were poor at that time in NHS laboratories and the attrition rate of those seeking alternative and better-paid employment would eventually contribute to a further loss of Student members.

By 1951, the excess of income was down to just £500 and Council reluctantly considered increasing the Student membership fees. During the same year, there was an 8% increase in overall membership numbers, with Student numbers remaining static, which translated to an increase in other grades and additional income for the Institute.

At this time, Council was giving much thought to purchasing larger premises on a long-term lease, with a view to having a stable location for the Registered Office. It hoped to achieve this without the need to take out a mortgage; this required having sufficient capital, which in 1951 was not available. Harry Barker never witnessed this ambition, although he played a major role in the financial preparations which finally resulted in the acquisition of 74 New Cavendish Street in May 1958, a few months after his death.

***

Sidney James Denyer (1894–1951) was the architect of the transition of the PBLAA into the Institute of Medical Laboratory Technology. Sidney Denyer commenced his career in 1908 at the laboratories of the Clinical Research Association in London, and he joined the PBLAA on its creation in 1912. Two years later, he volunteered for military service in the First World War, joining the Royal Army Medical Corps, and, after rapid promotion, was put in charge of a mobile laboratory at the front, where he served throughout the duration of the war.

On his discharge from the Army, in 1919, Denyer was appointed to the laboratories at the Ministry of Agriculture at Weybridge in Surrey. This was a significant period in his career as he would have come into contact with Albert Norman who had moved to the Weybridge laboratory in 1913. His involvement with the PBLAA was certainly a consequence and he soon took on various roles in the London Division before becoming a Council member in 1924. He served on Council with only one short break until 1936 when he was elected Honorary Secretary of the PBLAA, a role he continued to fulfil through to the formation of the Institute in 1942, becoming its first Honorary Secretary.

The six years up to the formal beginning of the Institute were probably the most onerous and difficult times for any Institute officer, starting with the growing dissatisfaction of the PBLAA membership in the late 1930s, and many calls for change, through to the endless legal and procedural work involved in giving birth to the IMLT. All this was undertaken during the darkest days of the Second World War in Britain, while continuing his employment and moving to Yorkshire.

Earlier, Denyer had been elected Vice President of the PBLAA in 1931–2 (at that time the appointment was for one year only). In 1934 he was one of the principal figures in the creation of *The Monthly Bulletin*, in collaboration with F R Chopping and C E Layng, and was its first Editor until his appointment as Honorary Secretary in 1936.

In 1944, Council decided to appoint a full-time General Secretary, largely on the advice of Sidney Denyer. He had already signalled that his honorary post was inappropriate for the increasing role of the new Institute. On his retirement as Honorary Secretary, he was elected a Vice Chairman of Council and was elected as a Vice President of the Institute in 1945, in recognition of his immense contributions.

Following his move to Wakefield in Yorkshire, in 1940, Sidney Denyer soon became involved in local activities as a keen cricketer in the Wakefield League, and also in politics, being elected to Wakefield City Council in 1949. On his death, he was honoured not only by his Institute colleagues but also by the Lord Mayor of Wakefield at his funeral in Wakefield Cathedral on 30 October 1951.

Chapter 10

Advent of the National Health Service
A Third Way For The Institute

The post-war 1940s were years of social and political change. In addition to introducing the NHS, Britain nationalised its coal industry and celebrated the wedding of Princess Elizabeth to Philip Mountbatten. Elsewhere in the world, Henry Ford died, the first airplane flew faster than the speed of sound, and partition of the Indian subcontinent resulted in the creation of an independent India and the new, independent state of Pakistan.

In the period following the passing of the *National Insurance Act (1946)* and the impending introduction of a National Health Service (NHS), the Institute increasingly became involved in the issues of salaries and conditions for medical laboratory workers. This has to be viewed in light of the fact that one of the key principles of the founding of the Institute was that it should not act as a trades union and was prohibited in doing so by the terms of its own Memorandum of Association.

This fact, however, did not prevent the Institute from pursuing a very active campaign to be involved in negotiating salary and conditions for its members, and to seek an official position for itself in this respect. Although the trades unions were active in official discussions, their position was at this time neither dominant nor fully recognised.

The mechanism to set salary levels for medical laboratory staff, prior to the introduction of the NHS, was the Recommendations of the Joint Committee on Salaries and Wages (Hospital Staff), which set the benchmark. The Institute was proactive in responding to these Recommendations, which had not been particularly well received. In addition, there was also another set of rules for the remuneration of laboratory staff employed by municipal authorities, published through the Schemes and Conditions for Local Government Officers.

The Institute, conscious of the limitations imposed on it by its Articles of Association, sought to maximise its efforts to achieve a better outcome for its members by setting up a meeting with the four trades unions – the Association of Scientific Workers (AScW), the Confederation of Health Service Employees (COHSE), the National Association of Local Government Officers (NALGO) and the National Union of Public Employees (NUPE) – believed to be most supportive of its aims. The trades unions agreed with the Institute in seeking to establish a Negotiating Committee for Laboratory Technicians, which would operate between the Joint Committee on Salaries and Wages and the Trade Unions. The first meeting of the new committee took place on 7 November 1946, at which it was requested that the Institute be represented by an observer at its future meetings.

The Institute was now involving itself increasingly in a role hitherto not undertaken by its predecessor. Earlier, the PBLAA had sought to develop in two areas: first, to support the professional interests of its members through scientific activities, and second, to establish an examination system to gain recognisable qualifications and standards of practice. The Institute was now embarking on a third role, that of political positioning and representation. This development caused alarm and concern among some Council members who believed that this role should be strictly limited.

The Institute had already worked to establish good relations with the Ministry of Health, pending the advent of the NHS, and had been consulted on several issues. Council realised that its operational activities were increasing rapidly and it was proposed that larger premises and additional staff would be required to support the Registered Office.

***

On 31 August 1947 the Institute moved its headquarters to new premises on the fourth floor of 76 Brewer Street, London W1. The annual rental was £350, for one large room, which was divided to form two offices. Although this was an improvement on the old accommodation, the move had been hastened on notice to quit from 12 Buckingham Street. This move was once again only temporary, as additional work and the recruitment of three additional staff required Council to take on a suite of offices located at 9 Harley Street, London W1, above the headquarters of the British Tar Industry. This was at the 'other end' of Harley Street, distant from that part of the thoroughfare popularly associated with prestigious private medical consulting rooms; nonetheless, the rent was now more than £1000 per year.

To put this in perspective, the annual subscription for a Fellow at the time was two guineas (£2.10), for an Associate it was one and half guineas (£1.57) and for a Student it was 10 shillings (£0.50), and more than one-third of the total membership of 3000 were students – this meant that the new rent represented a significant proportion of income. The Institute took up residence on 17 December 1949 and remained there for more than eight years.

A further consolidation of the central office function was the appointment of Richard Lavington to the full-time post of General Secretary, on 1 March 1948. There was another staff appointment of significance at this time, when Michael Lewis was recruited as an Administrative Officer. Michael Lewis joined the Institute after military service in the Second World War, having taken part in the D-Day landings. Council recorded that following his appointment there had been a vast improvement in record-keeping at the Registered Office. He spent the rest of his working life at the Institute and was well known to many Council members for his meticulous detailing of the financial arrangements, especially those associated with the Triennial conferences.

When the NHS formally came into existence in July 1948, the arrangements whereby the Institute had an observer role on the Joint Negotiating Committee for Medical Laboratory Technicians ceased to exist, and the committee was disbanded.

***

The Whitley Council for Health Service Employees now took responsibility for negotiating and setting pay scales for all NHS staff. The Institute immediately sought representation on the body's Functional Council, but had its applications rejected repeatedly by the Staff Side representatives.

The Institute's Council was determined to gain representation and agreed to make a direct approach to the Minister of Health, Aneurin Bevan. The matter was passed to the Staff Side of Whitley Functional Council 'B', and its response suggested that the Institute should hold a referendum of the membership to ascertain the level of support for its role. This was carried out and an overwhelming level of support was received for Council to continue its quest.

Eventually, the Secretary of the Staff Side replied that a meeting could be arranged between Institute representatives and the Chairman of Council 'B'; however, it is likely that this was only agreed after some pressure from the Association of Clinical Pathologists and the Pathological Society, whose members sat on a Pathology Committee at the Ministry of Health.

The issue continued into 1950, at which point Council decided that, as no progress towards an agreed outcome had been reached, it would inform Professor Bedson, chairman of the Pathology Committee, of its intention to have the situation raised in Parliament, through two MPs who were sympathetic to the Institute's aspirations.

The whole affair was effectively brought to a standstill on the appointment of the Cope Committee to examine the status of health service 'auxiliary staff', a group in which medical laboratory technicians were included.

***

Eight committees were set up by the Minister for Health to begin work on establishing a system of national regulation of educational criteria for non-medical staff working in the NHS who were working with or influencing the care of patients. A further key objective was to establish a statutory register of those practising in their respective professions. The committees were named after Vincent Zachary Cope, an eminent London surgeon, who chaired all eight committees. He was said to have greatly revered the work of Almroth Wright during the early years of his career.

At the time the Cope Committee was set up to examine the status of medical laboratory technicians, a total of 3195 members were registered with the Institute, including Students, which represented about a quarter of the 13,000 staff included in the Medical Auxiliaries category. The others included physiotherapists, the largest group with 4019 members, and radiographers with 2444. The others were almoners, occupational therapists, chiropodists, dieticians, remedial gymnasts and speech therapists. This grouping of professions has continued to be used for statutory registration up to the present day, probably more for the convenience of government than the best interests of the professions represented.

The Institute was requested to respond to a detailed questionnaire from the Committee as part of its research into the background to the role of medical laboratory technicians. Albert Norman, the Institute Chairman, represented Council in the discussions.

The Institute Council was concerned by the likelihood that the purpose of the exercise was the creation of a State Register of practitioners, and the possible undermining of the Institute as the professional qualifying body for medical laboratory technicians. However, on publication of the Report of the Committee on Medical Auxiliaries in April 1951, the findings were that the system of training and qualification undertaken by the Institute was "generally suitable" for medical laboratory technicians in the NHS.

The overall provisions were that all persons qualified to work in the NHS should be eligible for entry on a State Register, and nobody should be appointed to a NHS post without being on that register.

A number of issues from the Cope Report were destined to affect medical laboratory technicians and the Institute far into the future. The profession would be referred to as a Medical Auxiliary in the NHS, and there was a recommendation that a 'National Register' of Medical Auxiliaries should be kept to inform employers in the NHS of qualified staff; in effect, the precursor to plans for a State Register.

Professor James Dible (formerly President of the Institute, 1938–1948) gave evidence to the Committee in 1949, as an official 'witness', and he stated that any release of students from the workplace to attend courses "was disruptive to the working of the department and should not be considered". There was poor recognition, in the report, of the need to improve students' knowledge of the underlying scientific basics in biology, chemistry and physics. The perception was that the work of medical laboratory technicians was solely practical and required an 'apprenticeship-type' training to develop skills and was best undertaken in the workplace under supervision.

Blood Transfusion Centre staff were regarded as separate from medical laboratory technicians with regard to their training and qualification. It was felt that blood transfusion technicians performed barely at Intermediate level due to their narrow work experience and training. Their only support came from the Association of Scientific Workers (AScW) union which believed that there should be a separate Institute Final examination for this group.

There was general accord that Institute examinations and qualifications were appropriate for medical laboratory technicians; however, there was a belief that Fellowship was not and should not be a prerequisite for senior and chief posts in the NHS. This greatly undermined the Institute as a statutory qualifying and registering body for those working in the NHS. It almost certainly formed the basis for the barriers placed before the Institute for many years by other professions in the NHS and government in its attempts to develop the skills of modern biomedical scientists and obtain recognition of their qualifications by the medical establishment, the academic world and the public at large.

The Association of Clinical Pathologists (ACP) gave advice to the Committee that "at a guess" there was need for about 5000 (medical laboratory technicians) and that the current rate of recruitment was adequate to meet the staffing demand.

***

The Institute and its membership were generally uncomfortable with the findings of the Cope Committee and this gave rise to similar dissatisfaction among the other 'Auxiliary' health professions, to the point that on 19 March 1953, the Minister of Health, Ian Macleod, announced in Parliament that statutory registration as outlined in the Cope Report would not be taken forward. He also stated that there would be new regulations to set out the required qualifications for medical auxiliaries to be employed in the NHS. These were published in The National Health Service Medical Auxiliaries Regulations, 1954.

The Institute was named as the appropriate qualifying body for medical laboratory technicians, the Final Examination being cited as the primary qualification, with the alternatives of a UK science degree or Associate membership of the Royal Institute of Chemistry – a satisfactory outcome for the Institute.

In 1954 it was announced, in Parliament, that a new Working Party would be set up to pursue the establishment of a Statutory Register for Auxiliary Health Professions. This time, with agreement in mind, representatives of the appropriate professional groups were sought and the Council appointed Albert Norman (Chairman) and Richard Lavington (General Secretary) as their nominees. This was the beginning of the long process, lasting more than five years, which resulted in the *Professions Supplementary to Medicine (PSM) Act, 1960* being put on the statute book.

***

A draft scheme for Statutory Registration had been put forward by the Department of Health in 1956, following numerous amendments, and the British Medical Association put forward two late amendments, which it stated would be necessary in order to gain medical acceptance of the scheme. At the Institute Council meeting in October 1959, chaired by R J Bromfield, there was much apprehension and debate pending publication of the Draft Bill on Statutory Registration.

Chapter 11

The Swinging Sixties

Driving Change in Education
and Science with Professional Regulation

Think of the 1960s and the city of Liverpool comes easily to mind, linked forever through an enduring association with comedy, popular music and football. The decade also saw Man's quest to conquer space intensify, and the successful landing, in 1969, of the Eagle in the Sea of Tranquility on the Moon. "A giant leap...", as Neil Armstrong said at the time, in the relatively few years since President John F Kennedy committed the United States to the lunar landing programme.

Developments in medicine and science in the late 1950s and early 1960s resulted in major changes to the work undertaken in medical laboratories, in the complexity, range and number of tests and investigations carried out. Alongside this situation, there was recognition among senior members of the profession, particularly those involved in teaching and on the Institute Council, that there should be a greater component of pure science in the education of medical laboratory technologists. There was a prevailing 'traditional view' among some that the Intermediate and Final examinations were still fit for purpose. However, this was not the opinion of government and its education advisors.

The 1960s also heralded a new era in the Institute's most senior officer appointments. Reginald Bromfield, on his retirement as Chairman of Council at the end of 1960, was the last Chairman from the cadre who had served on the Council of the PBLAA. His successor, William Valentine, who was first appointed to the Institute Council in 1943, represented a new breed of Institute chairmen who would oversee major changes in the education and qualification of medical laboratory technologists.

***

Reginald Bromfield was Chairman of the Institute from 1958 until the end of 1960. In 1958 he was elected a Vice President of the Institute and a member of the Pathological Society of Great Britain and Ireland. His laboratory career started at University College in London and in 1922 he moved to the Hospital for Sick Children, Great Ormond Street, where he assisted Dr David Nabarro in establishing the biochemistry laboratory. In 1929 he moved to the Hospital for Tropical Diseases, where he came close to losing his life when he contracted a virulent form of yellow fever. Bromfield recovered but a less fortunate colleague died from the same disease after taking a blood sample from him.

Reginald Bromfield's major contributions to the profession were his services to the PBLAA and the Institute. He joined the PBLAA in 1923 and was elected to Council in 1934, where he continued his membership after the formation of the Institute in 1942. Apart from his period as Chairman, he is best remembered for his editorship of the *The Laboratory Journal* and

Monthly Bulletin (the forerunner of *The Gazette* and *The Biomedical Scientist*). In 1946 he joined Albert Norman as assistant editor. Norman, who had been editor since the inception of the *The Laboratory Journal* in 1913, stepped down and, in 1950, Bromfield took over as editor, a role he continued to occupy until his retirement in 1966.

A most significant issue on which Reginald Bromfield guided Council to debate during his chairmanship was the draft legislation leading up to the establishment of a statutory register of medical laboratory technicians. A draft scheme was first circulated as early as 1956, following numerous minor amendments. The British Medical Association (BMA) then put forward two late amendments that would be necessary for medical acceptance.

Bromfield had to handle considerable debate and opposition by Council, in considering the much-changed draft, prior to the publication of a Draft Bill on Statutory Registration.

***

The Minister of Health had stated on 28 July 1959 that it was the intention of government to introduce the legislation at an early date – this was later included in the Queen's Speech, to be in the subsequent Parliamentary session of 1960.

The Institute Council eventually resolved "that the representatives (Bromfield, Lavington and Valentine) be empowered to discuss statutory registration with other interested parties (other professional societies), notwithstanding any resolutions of Council which have embodied objections to the scheme, and shall take such action as may appear to be expedient. A decision of the Council shall be necessary before opting out of the scheme".

The designation of Institute members in the new scheme also gave rise to much varied opinions, as the favoured term 'technologist' had been ignored by the Health Minister, leaving 'technician' as the description in official correspondence. Other suggestions of 'technical officer' and 'laboratory technical officer' were rejected in Council.

In 1962 a memorandum was issued by the Ministry of Health, defining the outcomes of the *Professions Supplementary to Medicine (PSM) Act 1960*, also announcing the initial list of medical laboratory technician registrants in 1961. A further significant announcement from the Ministry of Health gave discretionary powers to health authorities to grant time off with pay to students and junior medical laboratory technicians for the attendance at classes held during normal working hours, up to one working day per week. This was a landmark decision for a concession that had previously been vigorously resisted by government officials and pathologists.

***

The Medical Laboratory Technicians Register commenced in 1963 and statutory registration became a condition of employment in qualified grades in the NHS from 1964. In the same year, the first register of Medical Laboratory Technicians was published and Mr W H Valentine (then Institute Chairman) was appointed Chairman of the Medical Laboratory Technicians (MLT) Board of the Council of Professions Supplementary to Medicine (CPSM).

The Board comprised 13 members, seven of whom were required to be members of the relevant profession, chosen to represent the members of that profession and their alternates. It was stipulated that there should be at least one member who was resident and practising in Scotland and in Wales. The other members included an expert in professional education and five medical members including one to represent Scottish interests.

Clearly, this gave a 'working majority' to the professional representatives of each Board, despite every effort by the medical profession, with the support of the BMA, to gain authority over the ethics and training of the professions supplementary to medicine. However, the ultimate control of the registration process resided with the Privy Council.

Initially, seven of the 14 professional representatives and their alternates on the MLT Board were Institute Council members, which rose to nine at the time of the first election of representatives in July 1964. There had been much anxiety and fear within the Institute that the new statutory registration process would undermine and diminish its purpose and functions. The outcome of the level of representation achieved soon allayed this apprehension with a strong constituent of Council officers, albeit each acting as an independent member of the MLT Board.

The functions of the Institute and the MLT Board became mutually beneficial. The interests of the MLT Board were solely with the qualifications required for registration, which allowed the Institute to move its focus to becoming a professional body for qualified members and to develop post-registration courses and qualifications at a higher level. The move away from a student-focused qualifying body was an important step in raising the profile and status of the Institute.

A feature of the PSM Act required that each professional Board produced an annual register, a function previously undertaken by the Institute, in 1952 and 1956, at considerable expense. In addition, a list of laboratories approved for the training of medical laboratory technicians was an MLT Board requirement. Both of these, and their associated costs, subsequently became a responsibility of the Board.

A further duty of the MLT Board was the establishment of a code of conduct and a disciplinary procedure. A Statement of Infamous Conduct was also issued later in 1965. The Institute had published a 'Code of Professional Conduct' in 1957, which was approved at that year's Annual General Meeting and enshrined in an addition to the Articles of Association. As no actions had been effected under this code, it was rescinded in favour of the MLT Board code in 1975 as it was felt that most of the Institute's members were also registered with the MLT Board. A further change occurred in 1982, when the Institute published a new 'Code of Professional Conduct', approved by Council, which better reflected the working environment of the time.

The Council for Professions Supplementary to Medicine was replaced by the Health Professions Council on 1 April 2002.

***

William Henry Valentine became Chairman of Council at the beginning of 1961, his period of office and personal contributions being of major significance in the development of the Institute and to the profession. Mr Valentine, as he was known to most of his Institute colleagues, and Bill to only to a small group of his longest associates, had already served at every level.

He was co-founder and later chairman of the Exeter branch, chairman of Midland region and was elected to Council in 1943. He was appointed a Vice President in 1960 and received an OBE in 1968.

During his time on Council, Valentine was a member of the General Purposes Committee (later the Executive Committee) and the Examinations Board. In 1956 he conducted the first Intermediate examination to be held outside the United Kingdom, in Nigeria. He also supervised the first Institute examinations to be held in Uganda and Mauritius. In addition to these roles, he served as Honorary Editor of *The Gazette* from 1951 until 1960, after having been Assistant Editor of *The Laboratory Journal*.

In an article in *The Gazette* in January 1964, he stated that he regarded his chairmanship of the 1962 Golden Jubilee Conference, held on 11–18 August, in Edinburgh, to be one of the most pleasurable tasks that he had undertaken during his period as Chairman of Council. This Conference celebrated 50 years of the Institute and the PBLAA, and was made all the more notable by the attendance of Albert Norman.

William Valentine oversaw the creation of two new Institute positions in 1962. In January of that year, the first Deputy General Secretary, John K Fawcett, was appointed. This was to be a very timely decision as Richard Lavington, the General Secretary, was taken ill soon after and John Fawcett very ably took over the full role until Lavington's return, several months later. However, John Fawcett maintained a key role as Lavington then worked reduced hours until his retirement, after which Fawcett was promoted to become General Secretary in April 1970.

The second position was that of Honorary Librarian, bestowed on John Mercer. A small collection of books had been accrued over the previous decade and, as a result of John Mercer's dedicated efforts over the next 50 years, this figure now stands at more than 1500 titles, including many first editions and rare volumes.

William Valentine continued to serve on Council long after his tenure as Chairman. He had been a member of the Joint Standing Pathological Committee and, in 1963, on the formation of the Standing Joint Committee with the College of Pathologists, began more than 20 years of service on this committee. As a Vice President he also sat on the Finance and the Publicity and Services committees throughout the 1970s. In addition, Mr Valentine completed 10 years as Chairman of the MLT Board, from its formation until his retirement in July 1972. At his last meeting, his period of office was described by Thomas Lansley as of "inestimable value to the Board, the profession and the Health Service".

***

Guy Pascoe was born in 1912, the same year in which the PBLAA was formed; therefore, it is most appropriate that his life and work should be so closely associated with the Association and Institute. He joined the PBLAA in 1930 after beginning his career at the Department of Bacteriology and Experimental Pathology of Guy's Hospital in London. In 1934 he moved to become senior technician in the Virol Pathological Research Laboratories – Virol was a commercial nutrition supplement based on malt extract.

In 1939, at the outbreak of the Second World War, after having moved to Park Hospital in Davyhulme, near Manchester, he was then attached to the Military Hospital in Davyhulme, where he worked throughout the duration of hostilities. He returned to London after the war and, after a short period at North Middlesex Hospital in charge of the microbiology section, was appointed chief technician of the pathology department at Prince of Wales Hospital, Tottenham, in 1947. He continued here until his retirement.

Guy Pascoe was actively involved in branch affairs, particularly the London branch, which he joined in 1945, and later served as Chairman for eight years. He was elected a National member of Council in 1952 and served on the General Purposes and Membership committees, and as the first chairman of the newly formed Finance Committee.

One of Guy Pascoe's lasting legacies is the Coat of Arms granted to the Institute in 1960. He was instrumental in the complex and protracted negotiations with the College of Arms, which finally resulted in the design we still recognise and use today.

He was appointed Vice Chairman of Council in 1961 and succeeded William Valentine as Chairman in 1964, with Thomas Lansley as Vice

Chairman. A quotation from the *Annual Report 1964* states "The Institute was thus assured of secure and balanced judgement in its direction, continuing the tradition of statesmanship, characteristic of its previous chairman, Mr W H Valentine".

Guy Pascoe had long been interested in education and training and he was involved in the introduction of classes for the Intermediate examination at the Prince of Wales Hospital in conjunction with Tottenham Technical College (he is remembered with affection by one of the authors [AJH] who attended this course).

In June 1964, Guy Pascoe attended the conference of the International Association of Medical Laboratory Technologists (IAMLT) in Lausanne, Switzerland, which commemorated the 10th anniversary of the formation of the IAMLT. He was elected to the Council of the IAMLT, replacing Richard Lavington, who had served on the Council since its inception and was retiring at the end of his term of office. Guy Pascoe became a prominent figure in the IAMLT, was elected President at the Chicago Congress in 1976, served until 1978 and then became the first Executive Director until 1980.

Guy Pascoe is remembered as a great ambassador and diplomat for the Institute at home and abroad. He also had a keen interest in the history of the profession and served as chairman of the Historic Section until shortly before his death in 1991.

***

The final month of 1964 marked the end of an era with the death of Albert Norman, aged 82, on 22 December. Although he had retired 12 years earlier he had continued to serve on the Institute's Council, attending a meeting only a few weeks before his death.

A Service of Remembrance was held at the Church of St Bartholomew-the-Less, situated within St Bartholomew's Hospital, on 19 February 1965. This was attended by Mrs Norman, Council members, Vice Presidents, including John McLean, then aged 90, and many members who had come to celebrate the life and achievements of the founder of the first professional organisation for non-medical staff employed in pathology laboratories.

The memory of Albert Norman would be perpetuated by the Albert Norman Memorial Lecture, given at each Triennial Conference (now Congress). In 1967, Council established a trust fund of £1000 to cover the expenses of a guest lecturer at each conference.

***

The administration associated with the increasing business of the Institute required Council to seek additional accommodation at the Registered Office. During the period of occupancy of offices at 74 New Cavendish Street, membership numbers had increased from 7000 in 1958 to more than 12,000 in 1965. In the days just before Christmas 1965, an agreement for the purchase of a lease for 12 Queen Anne Street, near Harley Street, in London, was completed; these premises are a short distance from the previous address. The transfer of all the office functions was completed and the new office opened officially in April 1966.

The arrangements for this move were to cause financial concerns for Council. The sale of the remaining term of the leasehold on 74 New Cavendish Street fell through at a late stage. The Institute was left with a shortfall and little prospect of completing a sale during a credit squeeze with a static property market. This resulted in the Institute bearing large interest costs in servicing a bank overdraft to meet the cost of the new lease.

There had been a realisation in Council that revenues were not meeting the increasing costs of activities, and, in 1965, a decision was taken to raise the membership fees for the first time since 1947. The increases, operable from 1 January 1966, were large in percentage terms, nearly doubling the fees, but were still less than most other similar professional bodies. In modern times, it is unthinkable that fees had been left unchanged for 18 years – a situation that no subsequent Treasurer has allowed to be repeated.

***

Thomas Stewart Lansley joined the PBLAA in 1939, prior to the outbreak of the Second World War, beginning his medical laboratory career at St Mary Abbots Hospital in Kensington in 1938. His career was put on hold when he joined the RAF Volunteer Reserve in 1940 and was sent to Southern Rhodesia (now Zimbabwe) to train as a pilot. He succeeded in this respect and on his return to England undertook further training to become a flying instructor. He logged more than 1400 hours flying during his war service.

On return to civilian life in 1946 he resumed his scientific work at the London County Council Laboratory Service before a number of appointments in North London hospitals, including a spell at the Prince of Wales Hospital, Tottenham, where Guy Pascoe also worked.

In 1955, Tom Lansley was appointed senior technician at East Ham Memorial Hospital, where he remained until his retirement as senior chief medical laboratory scientific officer in 1983.

In the early 1950s, Tom was a keen member of the London branch Biochemical Discussion Group (along with a young John Fawcett). He later joined the branch committee and became chairman in 1957.

Tom Lansley was elected as a National Council member in 1958 and was elected Vice Chairman in 1964 to serve during the chairmanship of Guy Pascoe. He succeeded Pascoe to become Chairman of the Institute from 1 January 1967, and his three-year period of office encompassed some of the most challenging legislation to affect members of the Institute and the biomedical science profession.

The portfolio of Institute appointments held by Tom Lansley is unique and exceeds that of anyone, including Albert Norman. He served on every committee of Council, the majority as chairman, from 1958 until 1982. From 1963 to 1975 he was the Institute's advisor to the Whitley Council and regularly reported on the many developments in this respect to Council and in articles in *The Gazette*, explaining the implications affecting biomedical scientists working in the NHS. Notably, he also served on the MLT Board from 1962, and took over as chairman from W H Valentine in 1972 until retiring in 1982.

Tom Lansley's role in changing the direction of education in biomedical science was fundamental to the eventual achievement of a degree-based entry to the profession. His role in developing the National Certificate programme across the United Kingdom is without equal. Between 1966 and 1977 he served on and chaired the Joint Committee for Ordinary and Higher National

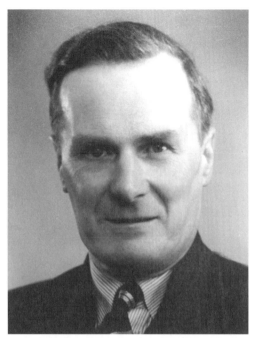

Reginald J Bromfield

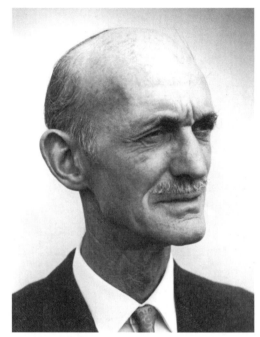

William H Valentine

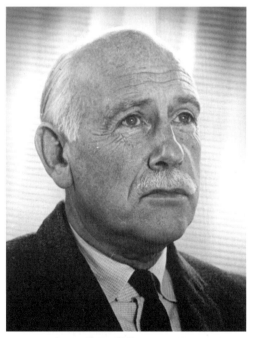

Guy C Pascoe

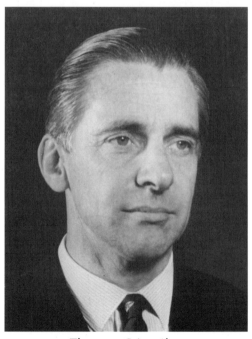

Thomas S Lansley

Certificates for England and Wales, also the Scottish Joint Committee for National Certificates and Diplomas, and was the Institute representative on the Irish National Committee for Medical Laboratory Sciences.

Tom Lansley had a special ability to speak on the most complex issues and was able to relate a clear explanation to any audience. He had been asked by both his predecessors to address annual general meetings to explain special resolutions and developments on the future of education.

A further example of the scope of his interests and foresight is recorded in an article entitled 'Help from a Computer', published in *The Gazette* in May 1968. In his article, Lansley reviewed a study on 'Computer Use in Pathology Laboratories', carried out at the Nuffield Medical Data Processing Unit, stating: "The value of the study lies in the preliminary analysis of pathology work, record-keeping and clerical functions, and in the help it gives in understanding the relevance of computer facilities to laboratory work". This was well over decade before computers appeared in most laboratories.

***

The principal concern of Council in 1967 was the decision by the Minister of Health and Secretary of State for Scotland to set up a committee "to consider the future organisation and development of hospital scientific and technical services in National Health Service hospitals and the broad pattern of staffing required and to make recommendations". Sir Solly Zuckerman was appointed to chair the committee, and the subsequent report is often referred to as the Zuckerman Report.

The report entitled 'Hospital Scientific and Technical Services: Report of the Committee 1967–68 (1968)' was published in December 1968, less than a year from the committee's first meeting. Evidence was received from many individuals and organisations including the Institute – Dr A D Farr gave a detailed account of the Zuckerman Report in *Learn, that you may improve*, published by Denley Instruments in 1982.

Council published its response to the report in March 1969 in a pamphlet, entitled 'Comments on the Report of the Hospital Scientific and Technical Services Committee', addressed to the Secretary of State for Social

Services and the Secretary of State for Scotland. The comments were included under eight headings: i) Consultation, ii) Hospital Scientific Service, iii) Career Structure, iv) Training, Qualification and Promotion, v) Technical Aides, vi) Technical and Scientific Officers, vii) Other Bodies, and viii) Future Planning.

There was criticism of the "superficial report" and the unacceptably limited representation of the medical laboratory technician contingent (represented by the Institute), the members of which comprised more than one-third of hospital scientific and technical staff. "The Institute earnestly hopes that the Ministers will compensate in their subsequent consultations for the lack of balance in the constitution of the committee by seeking the advice and help available from the professional societies representing the major areas in the scientific and technical services".

Concern was expressed on the inclusion of authority over training of staff in the response, stating: "It (the Institute) is convinced, however, that the influence of the Department and of the National Scientific Councils on training should be limited to an advisory capacity".

In commenting on the proposals for changes in the career structure, the response states: "The Institute welcomes the intention to introduce an open-ended career structure but notes that the implementation of the recommendations of the Hospital Scientific and Technical Services Committee may not necessarily lead to this objective. A separation into four discrete classes, instead of a career ladder with stepping off stages according to the level of qualification attained, would be no answer to the problem for which the committee was expected to find solutions".

On future planning, the response reads: "The Institute of Medical Laboratory Technology expects that it will be asked in due course to appoint representatives on the working parties that the Ministers may set up to advise on the planning of the particular services and on the integration of the present staff into a new structure. The Institute also should be invited to nominate members of the proposed regional scientific advisory committees. The Institute proposes that the various interested parties should meet together in the near future to survey laboratory functions on a broader and more representative basis than the Hospital Scientific and Technical Services

Committee has done, so that conclusions may be reached objectively".

The underlying objective of the Zuckerman Report had been to establish a single grading spine for Hospital Scientific Service staff in the NHS. There was a less than enthusiastic response from medical laboratory workers, and strong criticism of the proposals from the Institute and the CPSM, citing numerous inaccuracies and the clear inconsistency with the Scientific Civil Service (on which the proposals were modelled). In the lengthy period since the publication of Zuckerman, the Fulton report had reshaped the Civil Service grades and the Institute strongly lobbied the Department of Health to reconsider the proposals originally put forward to be aligned with those recommended by Fulton.

The Institute continued to press the case for a unified staffing structure, in policy statements published in 1972 and 1974, against a background of increasing professional concerns of the Zuckerman proposals, which had not yet been implemented.

The subsequent and long-running divisions created following this report went on for many years and can be viewed objectively as the first of a number of damaging actions by a succession of governments on a group of highly qualified and regulated staff performing a vital service in support of the diagnosis and treatment of disease in the National Health Service.

The failure to deliver an acceptable and effective outcome caused the issues to remain unresolved such that in 2011, the manifestations of the latest initiative, entitled *Managing Scientific Careers*, is now the subject of uncertainty and a long-running process of discussion.

***

The Institute, during the chairmanship of Thomas Lansley, had to contend with a further political initiative that impinged on educational policy. In May 1967 the Secretary of State for Education and Science invited the National Advisory Council on Education for Industry and Commerce to review the national pattern and organisation of technician courses and examinations, including those leading to 30 various national certificates and several national diplomas in England and Wales. In 1969, a committee under the chairmanship of Dr H L Haslegrave, issued its report, recommending the establishment of a Technical Education Council (TEC).

A parallel review also took place in Scotland, under the chairmanship of Sir Edmund Hudson, culminating in the announcement of the establishment of the Scottish Technician Education Council (SCOTEC) in 1970.

The Institute gave evidence to both reviews, and on publication of the Haslegrave Report expressed its reservations of the proposals to the Secretary of State, Margaret Thatcher.

The outcome of the recommendations was the transfer of responsibility for all technician courses previously within the national certificates and diplomas grouping, to be taken over by the respective TECs. The Institute continued a dialogue with the Secretary of State and members of her department, as Council was particularly concerned about Department of Education plans to pass control of courses to TEC before it was formally established and to ensure that the Institute gained representation to the TEC structure.

Chapter 12

The Institute in the 1970s and 1980s

Organisational Change, Computers, Confrontation, and a Strong Presidential Voice

In the 1970s, floppy disks first saw the light of day, Microsoft was founded, Sydney Opera House opened, the movie Star Wars was released and Louise Brown, the first test tube baby, was born. The 1980s erupted at Mount St Helens, the Prince of Wales married Lady Diana Spencer, the Space Shuttle Discovery embarked on its maiden voyage and Ronald Reagan handed executive power to George Bush, who became the 41st President of the United States.

The 1970s witnessed major advances in medical treatment, with heart and lung transplantation often in the headlines. In the diagnostic field, computerised axial tomography (CAT) scanning was having an impact, and in the medical laboratory the introduction of automated analytical equipment in biochemistry and haematology was increasing, limited only by the financial constraints of the national economy.

The decade commenced against a backdrop of major change in the management of the NHS in the United Kingdom. A plan to decentralise the management of healthcare to 80 area health authorities, which would be responsible for managing an integrated health service of district hospitals and community services, was scheduled for implementation in 1974. Of more direct interest to the Institute and its members was continuing concern about the implementation of the Zuckerman Report.

In 1970, there were three significant personnel changes at the Institute: first, the election of Walter Finch as Chairman from 1 January, to succeed Thomas Lansley; second, the retirement of Richard Lavington after 22 years in office as General Secretary; and third, the appointment of John Fawcett as the new General Secretary, supported with the unanimous approval of Council. The appointment of Fawcett, who had served as Deputy General Secretary since 1962, would herald a number of organisational changes in the administrative functions of the Registered Office and, more importantly, the Committee structure of Council.

***

An Extraordinary General Meeting, chaired by Walter Finch, was held at the London School of Hygiene and Tropical Medicine on 21 November 1970. The purpose was to announce a special resolution that Council would put forward to amend the Memorandum of Association in relation to charity status.

Thomas Lansley introduced the topic by stating the need to obtain approval for the principle of charity status in order that the required amendment could be made to the Memorandum. It was explained that the Institute existed for the benefit of the community as a whole, a concept that had motivated the 14 original signatories to the Memorandum, and 28 years later it had become apparent that change would be worthwhile. Mr Lansley described the Institute's role and structure, with its activities at national, regional and branch level, which satisfied the Board of Trade and Charity Commissioners in fulfilling the criteria for charity status.

A sentence would be added to the Memorandum stating that the objects for which the Institute was established were to promote the science and to develop the practice of Medical Laboratory Technology for the public benefit. The resolution was approved and the Institute ultimately became a Charitable Body in 1971.

At that time it was estimated that an immediate annual saving of around £5000 would be made as a result of the change of status. At the current level of Institute activity, that saving probably runs into hundreds of thousands of pounds.

***

The retirement of Richard (Dickie) Lavington was marked by a special dinner held in the Fellows Restaurant at the Zoological Society of London, Regents Park, on 6 June 1970. This was attended by around 170 people, a feat Walter Finch described as "probably the most representative cross-section of the Institute that had ever been gathered together".

Richard Lavington was appointed General Secretary in 1948, following the damaging events occuring during the period of J M Signy's office. Dickie Lavington and Harry Barker helped rebuild the administrative and financial position of the Institute and, shortly before his retirement, Lavington was rewarded by his election as a Vice President at the 1970 Annual General Meeting, held in Manchester. He had previously been awarded Life Membership in 1956 and the Sims Woodhead Medal in 1969.

Walter Finch (1919–1991) spent his entire career working in London, with two spells at Miller General Hospital in Greenwich (1936–40 and 1944–46), moving to Queen Elizabeth Hospital, Bethnal Green, during 1940–44 and then to the London Jewish Hospital, Mile End (1946–54). He served for 10 years as a Chief Technician at the London Hospital Medical College before becoming a full-time lecturer at Paddington Technical College until his retirement in 1984.

Finch had been involved in Institute affairs on the London branch committee, serving as Treasurer, Chairman and representative to the South East region committee. However, the circumstances of his appointment to Council and his election as a Vice Chairman are rather bizarre and unusual.

The minutes of a Council meeting held at the Montague Hotel in Bloomsbury on 29 May 1965 showed that "In response to the Council's invitation, the London and South East region had nominated Mr W H Finch to fill the casual vacancy resulting from the death of Mr E C Clarke (the sitting regional Council member). This nomination would be considered at a special meeting of Council after the Annual General Meeting". He was subsequently elected, unopposed, as the South East region Council member at the Annual General Meeting of the Institute in 1966.

It is surprising, therefore, just two years after his official election to Council, that Walter Finch would be elected as Vice Chairman to succeed Thomas Lansley. The explanation being that an arrangement had been reached in case "a difficult situation may arise" whereby consideration of someone from outside of London "could not easily occupy the chair from 1970". Agreement was reached that George McKee from Belfast, who had originally been nominated as Vice Chairman in 1967 to succeed Lansley, would retire from Council at the Belfast Triennial Conference in August 1968. He was subsequently nominated to become a Vice President.

This may appear undemocratic by present-day standards, with the bias towards only appointing London-based Council members to higher office. However, the high cost and difficulties of lengthy travel at this time, together with the fact that paid leave of absence was unlikely to be granted, would appear to be valid factors in not appointing members residing outside the London region. George McKee may well have been a case in point. This, of course, all took place during an era before computer-based communication existed and long-distance telephone calls were still difficult.

It is perhaps not surprising that such manoeuvring occurred, when London-based, unelected members were coopted to Council committees, including the authoritative General Purposes Committee, rather than appointing a formally elected member of Council from outside of London. There may have been several reasons for these actions. The financial concerns of bringing elected Council members to London-based meetings from the regions was part of the frugal mentality that pervaded the Institute, probably as a result of its precarious financial position in its early years. The other, less-plausible reason was that the regional Council members' limited availability to attend London meetings on a regular basis would be obstructive to carrying out business in a timely manner.

It is understandable, therefore, that many members in the regions felt that the Institute was unduly focused in the capital. It is also hard to believe that these arrangements would have been accepted if more generally known to the membership as a whole. The subsequent review of the Council committee structure and a relaxation of financial constraints would regularise the composition of Council committees after 1971.

John Fincham was appointed Vice Chairman from January 1970, to succeed Walter Finch on his retirement. Once again, another unusual situation occurred when he stepped down in November 1970 in order to begin a Masters in Technology course in immunology. The outcome of this was the election of Frank Baker as Vice Chairman to take the chair in 1973, on the retirement of Walter Finch.

***

Since the formation of the PBLAA in 1912, Presidents had always been eminent pathologists. In the 1960s it is evident that tensions and conflicts of interest arose in relation to roles of the Chairman and President, and their relationships with the General Secretary. It took the statesmanship of W H Valentine, then Chairman, to address the situation at the Council meeting held at the Edinburgh Conference on 15 August 1962. Valentine stated: "It was evident that for several years there had been a tendency to modify the functions of Chairman and President. There was no need to go into the reason for this. The Chairman spoke of the difficulties created thereby and now wished to clear the air once and for all by making plain the constitutional position that the Chairman of the Institute is its chief executive officer: he is responsible to the Council and acts for the Council between Council meetings and he is vested with the authority of the Council.

"The President of the Institute is, by virtue of his office, Chairman of the Examinations Board and the Final Examining Body and he is responsible – within the limits of policy defined by the Council – for the conduct of the business of these bodies. The President does not make, or lay down, policy; his office, by tradition and in fact, has always been a consultative one. When there has been desire or need for consultation it has been a matter for the Chairman to consult or to delegate consultation. Executive decisions, apart from those matters indicated above, and policy decisions are matters for reference to the Chairman".

Valentine concluded that because the issue affected deeply the future life of the Institute, he wanted to restore and preserve the integrity of the office of Chairman. The Council affirmed the position without dissent.

Into the 1970s and the impetus for the Institute to seek autonomy from medical dependence was growing. This culminated in a Special Resolution, one of three presented at the 1974 Annual General Meeting held at the Sheffield Triennial Conference. This stated that "The Articles of Association of the Institute be amended by the deletion of the second paragraph of Article 64 and the substitution of the following: The Council may invite any Fellow of the Institute to act as President of the Institute. The President shall hold office for a period of three years and shall not be eligible for immediate re-election".

The effect of this and the other resolutions realised the aspiration that the office of Chairman and President would, in future, be combined following the retirement of the officers in post at that time. It was expected that the new President would normally be a practitioner of biomedical science. There would be no separate Chairman and Vice Chairman, but the immediate Past President would act as first deputy to the President, while the President Elect, chosen at least a year before the incumbent President retired, would be the second deputy.

The Special Resolutions were all passed with overwhelming majorities, paving the way for the first appointment of a President from the membership.

***

Frank Baker (1916–1999) holds the distinction of becoming, on 1 January 1976, the first non–medical President of the Institute, after having served previously as Chairman since 1973. He therefore served continuously for six years as Chairman and President, a feat that will not be equalled, under the Articles of Association. It is perhaps an irony that his predecessor, Professor George Dick, who had held office for eight years as the last medical President, was the most highly regarded during his long period of office, and many members saw his departure with much regret.

Frank Baker began his career in the laboratories of the London School of Hygiene and Tropical Medicine (LSHTM) in 1935 and, after a period at the Postgraduate Medical School in Hammersmith, returned to LSHTM in 1939. He was seconded to the Dunn School of Pathology in Oxford in 1940 but moved back to LSHTM as head technologist a year later. Between 1942 and 1945 he worked at the Agricultural Research Council Laboratory at Compton before returning again to LSHTM. His many posts brought him in contact with many eminent professors of bacteriology including Professors Topley, Wilson and Cruickshank, and on the formation of the NHS he was appointed as principal technologist in the Department of Pathology at the Brompton Hospital in London.

Frank Baker was elected to the Institute Council in 1966. He was a passionate believer that the Institute should be in control of its own direction and destiny, without reliance on the medical profession. He was elected Vice Chairman in 1971, following the resignation of W J Fincham, becoming Chairman from 1 January 1973. Frank Baker was a 'big personality' in all respects and was free in expressing his views. He was awarded an OBE in 1977 and elected a Vice President in 1980.

Biomedical science occupied much of his life and he spent many years lecturing to students of microbiology but he was also a prolific author and gained world acclaim as joint author of *Introduction to Medical Laboratory Technology*, first published in 1954, which continued for several editions and reprints. He published *Medical Microbiological Techniques* in 1962 and he also edited 14 volumes of the Laboratory Aides series.

A little known string to his impressive bow was his musical ability, performing as a saxophonist and leader of a small dance band, which played regularly in the West London area. With all his 'outside interests', Frank Baker would have received considerable support from the General Secretary in carrying out the duties of his offices.

***

Campaigning to move away from the designation of qualified staff as technicians had been pursued by the Institute and in Whitley Council by the Staff Side since 1956. They had argued that "the term technician has been used so freely as to have lost a good deal of its former significance". Within the NHS, the term has been applied to a variety of occupations, some of which had no syllabus of training, set examinations or professional qualification.

The Institute had issued a policy statement in 1972 entitled 'Staffing in Medical Laboratories' in which it described the increased scientific elements in both education and practice, adding to the skills and knowledge of members of the profession. Subsequently, there were several meetings with representatives of the Department of Health and Social Security, which had acknowledged the stance of the Institute and recommended that the Institute should communicate with the joint secretaries (Management and Staff Side) of the PTB Whitley Council. The Institute duly sent letters to the joint secretaries in 1973 setting out the case for change and seeking comparability with grades within the Scientific Civil Service, where staff were described in various grades of scientific officer.

***

The Triennial Conference of 1974, held in Sheffield on 10–17 August, was the setting for the instigation of the Institute changing its name. At the opening ceremony, the President, Professor George Dick, described the high level of qualifications of the profession and went on to state that the term of technician was no longer appropriate for members and that they should be known as scientific officers.

At the Annual General Meeting, held later on the same day, there was strong support voiced for the view that "the Institute should be forceful in introducing a more meaningful designation for the profession than medical laboratory technician". There was support for Council to seek the revised designation of scientific officer and that the name of the Institute should be changed to Institute of Medical Laboratory Sciences in support of changing the professional designation.

In 1975 the Institute changed its name to Institute of Medical Laboratory Sciences, and on 22 February 1978, at a meeting of Whitley Council PTB Committee A, it was agreed that the designation Medical Laboratory Technician be replaced by Medical Laboratory Scientific Officer for staff employed in NHS laboratories, and the term was adopted in medical laboratories across the country.

The term of office of Frank Baker as Chairman and President, with the great support of Professor Dick as President until 1975, heralded a major stride in the Institute's progress. One development, which undoubtedly benefited the President and Council, was the restructuring of the committees of Council and the reorganisation of the staff in the Registered Office.

***

The origins of the committee structure of the Institute were established at a meeting of the Council held on 7 April 1944. Mr G Harper, an experienced Council member from Birmingham, drew up a draft protocol for conducting the business of the Institute, which was approved and subsequently formed the basis for the first committees.

The main committee was the General Purposes and Membership Committee (GPC) and the others, Education, Editorial, Finance, Joint Standing Committee with The Pathological Society and The Association of Clinical Pathologists, and Overseas, were virtually subcommittees of the GPC. Of note, is that Albert Norman, then Chairman, sat on all but one of the committees and Eric C Chidwick, the chartered secretary who was instrumental in achieving the incorporation of the Institute, was a member of the Finance Committee. Subsequently, Finance and Membership became subcommittees of the GPC, Finance being re-established as a separate committee in 1957.

The committee structure evolved to meet the continuing growth and changing vocational needs of medical laboratory staff. By 1970, it was evident that, with the introduction of a radically new system of education and training, and a requirement for greater academic attainment, Council would need to meet these challenges with changes to its committee format.

The General Secretary, John Fawcett, prepared a memorandum on Committees that was presented at the Council meeting of 12 September 1970. The document examined the purpose of the committees and described proposals for a new structure, with the function and membership of each carefully detailed.

The new main committee of Council would be the Executive Committee, dealing with general policy, external relations (with other bodies) and administration. It would also have the authority to reconcile the policies of other committees. In 1971, the Chairman and Vice Chairman of Council would be ex-officio members, and five others would be elected by ballot. This committee superseded the GPC.

Council directed that the Executive Committee should oversee the introduction of six new committees covering the administrative requirements of Institute activity. The new committees would be Finance, Publicity and Services, Regulations, Fellowship, Examining Body (Final) and Medical Laboratory Management. Appointments to these new committees would only be from the elected members of Council, and most members would serve on at least two committees.

This change did away with the need to coopt members to Council committees, and ensured that all Council members, wherever they were based, would serve on Council committees.

This new order did come with additional costs to the administration of Council, and required all Council members to undertake more work and responsibility. All members would also now receive a full set of the minutes of all committee meetings, including those of which they were not members.

Under these revised arrangements, only elected Council members would participate on Council committees. The one exception to this was in relation to examination policy, when the views of members of the profession with relevant experience might be sought, despite the fact that they were not elected Council members. It was intended that the new structure would create more democracy and minimise the risk of committees vying against each other.

***

In March 1969, John Fawcett, then Deputy General Secretary, produced a detailed report for Council entitled 'Future Staffing Organisation'. A plan of the current staffing structure was presented, with alternatives based on the perceived changes envisaged to the business of the Institute following the changes taking place in education and examinations. Fawcett stated that there would be a reduction of work related to the administration of examinations as national certificates replaced the Intermediate and Final examinations. He forecast that financial savings could be made and the resources redirected into creating new posts with specific responsibilities in key areas.

A difficult period would ensue in the short term while the transition from Institute to national certificate examinations was completed. This period would demand additional staffing and expenditure to cope with the continuing organisation of Intermediate and Final examinations in addition to the increasing number of national certificates and higher examinations. The introduction of the Special examinations in seven different subjects had a particularly marked impact on the Registered Office, with problems arising from the processing of multiple-choice questions and the arrangement of oral examinations for candidates selected at fairly short notice. Fawcett advised that there was an imminent need for an additional examination assistant to address this extra work.

John Fawcett also highlighted the imminent retirement of the General Secretary (Richard Lavington) in 1970 and its implications. He described the need to redistribute responsibilities and the workload that had been shared by the General Secretary and his deputy within the Registered Office. He also stressed the need for a training programme and the strengthening of senior positions well before the date of retirement.

Following his appointment as General Secretary in 1970, John Fawcett soon established the changes that he had outlined in his 1969 report. The post of Deputy General Secretary was dropped and four new senior officer posts were created. The most significant was that of Finance Officer, which fulfilled the earlier recommendations of the auditors that an accountant should be appointed. There were concerns about the cost associated with filling this post with someone fully qualified, which resulted in the appointment of Mr J L Sidebottom, an experienced but less qualified person.

The post of Registration Officer to fulfil the functions of office manager and chief clerk was awarded to Mr Michael Lewis, a very experienced member of the existing staff. His duties would also include responsibility for membership details and record-keeping. During 1974, Michael Lewis was appointed Assistant General Secretary, a position he held until his retirement.

Another current member of staff, Miss Celia White, was appointed as Examinations Officer to be responsible for handling all the arrangements associated with the existing Final examinations and with the new national certificate schemes. This post was dropped in 1973, although Miss White remained on the staff. She celebrated 25 years' service at the Institute in 1978, and in recognition of this was presented with a clock by the President, Frank Baker.

Mr C Kenny, an Institute Fellow, was appointed to the fourth post, Information Officer, to undertake the work associated with *The Gazette*, including managing the advertising and assisting with editorial functions and publicity. In 1972, this post was also dropped and Mr Kenny returned to the laboratory at St Mary's Hospital in London.

These specific titles gave a new level of responsibility to their holders and provided the initial means to develop the services required to meet the increasing workload experienced in the Registered Office.

***

When Frank Baker was elected the last Chairman of the Institute to serve from 1973, Dennis Slade was elected Vice Chairman to serve the customary period of three years. Following the decisions to make the changes that facilitated the election of Frank Baker to serve as the first non-medical President from

January 1976, Dennis Slade had completed his office as Vice Chairman and was coopted back on to Council. He was then announced as the President Elect and had a further period of 'waiting in the wings' before becoming President in January 1979 on the retirement of Frank Baker.

Dennis Slade joined the Institute of Medical Laboratory Technology on leaving the Royal Army Medical Corps in 1948. He achieved Fellowship in 1955 and went on to become Chief Technician in haematology in the Area Laboratory, Musgrove Park Hospital, Taunton. He then moved to the Royal United Hospital in Bath, becoming Principal Technician in 1975. He was a member of the Exeter branch from 1953, moving to the Bristol branch in 1955, and was elected to Council in 1964 as the regional member for the South West.

Dennis Slade had considerable experience as a trades union representative, having served on area health service committees since 1954 and been a member of the Medical Laboratory Technicians and NHS National Advisory Committees since 1955. In his workplace he had been a member of the Hospital Joint Consultative Committee and chairman of the Staff Side for many years.

This experience proved to be most valuable during his term as President from 1979. During the previous years there had been mounting unrest among staff in NHS laboratories concerning pay and conditions, and Slade, having been involved in trades union discussions was very aware of the prevailing situation.

***

For many years the Institute had a presence at meetings of the Whitley Council Professional and Technical Staffs B (PTB) Committee A, where discussions concerning members working in NHS medical laboratories took place. This presence was as observers but also provided the opportunity to act as advisors, always aware of the Institute's status as a professional body under the terms of the Articles of Association.

There had been tensions in the relationship with trades unions representing medical laboratory staff but the Institute was always careful to recognise its non-union function and symbiotic role in supporting staff and management in achieving agreement. Experiences and situations in the late 1970s tested this stance to breaking point, especially when the unions proposed industrial action by their members, many of whom were also Institute members. A critical situation resulted following the widely publicised call to restrict out-of-hours working in pursuance of a pay claim.

This presented a dilemma for some Institute members who believed that the professional body should be bolder and more representative of members' interests; however, those same members did not wish to join a trades union in order to have their views represented because they were not prepared to take part in industrial action. When the membership had such difficulties in their relationship with the Institute, it is hardly surprising that society in general did not fully understand its position.

The Institute had to make a statement of its position and issued a Press Release on 13 March 1980.

Industrial Action in the Medical Laboratory Service

The continuing industrial dispute between trades unions and management in the medical laboratory service was discussed at a recent meeting of the Council of the Institute of Medical laboratory Sciences, when it was emphasised that professional responsibility for the well-being of patients must be the first concern of professional staff, however just the cause of an industrial dispute.

The industrial action by some NHS medical laboratory scientific officers, in the form of restricting services outside of normal contractual hours, began last November (1979) and still continues. The dispute results from a claim for increased payment for these duties. The Institute of Medical Laboratory Sciences regrets that the dispute, instead of being resolved, has become more complex. It is willing to use its role as consultant to both the management and staff sides of the PTB Whitley Council with the object of restoring the service.

The Institute deplores any situation developing, whatever its cause, which results in industrial action. Nevertheless, the Institute recognises that there are diverse views within the profession and that many of its members face a substantial dilemma in reconciling their professional responsibilities with the call for industrial action. It is important that the professional responsibilities accepted by registered medical laboratory scientific officers are not compromised during the industrial dispute. The profession has a vocational responsibility to sick people, and its members have to make their personal decisions in that light. Even if there is an irreconcilable conflict between professional responsibility and trades union loyalties, members of the profession can never properly take action that would endanger patients and put their lives at risk; such action would be inconsistent with professional ethics.

The Institute does not seek to impose a view on the merits of each side of the current dispute but, while it lasts, it expects medical laboratory scientists to act in accordance with their professional responsibilities.

It is not surprising that erroneous interpretations of this statement soon appeared in the daily press. An article followed in *The Daily Telegraph* headlined 'Lab staff's Institute attacks unethical industrial action'. In a published response, John Fawcett stated that "Contrary to the criticism of one side that readers might have inferred from your headline, we (the Institute) would do everything possible to bring both sides together in the interests of patients, the medical laboratory service and those who provide it".

***

Any organisation that seeks to grow and improve its position is going to come into an inevitable position of competitive conflict with others who view it as a new threat to their existing status. When two of the most significant developments in the history of the Institute occurred in quick succession, namely the change of title to Institute of Medical Laboratory Sciences in 1975, and the inauguration of Mr F J Baker as the first non-medical President in 1976, there was a reaction from a section of the medical establishment and subsequently from government health departments.

The Institute was constantly aware that health departments embarked on matters affecting the profession without reference to the appropriate body. One such situation came to a head in 1976 when Institute representatives met with health department officials to discuss post-HNC qualification training for the Special Examination, and were told that decisions about this training would be restricted and employing authorities would not be encouraged to grant further release for such courses. This was also part of a strategy by health departments to make recommendation to the Management Side of Whitley Council that Fellowship of the Institute, or any other post-HNC qualification, was not necessary for promotion to Senior, Chief, Senior Chief and Principal grade posts.

It transpired that the Department of Health in England (DHSS) had taken advice from its consultant advisors, including directors of the Blood Transfusion Service and Public Health Laboratory Service, who stated that no more than 25% of medical laboratory scientists should require post-HNC training or qualification.

The DHSS attempted to seek the agreement of the Institute to some modification of these arrangements. The Institute stood its ground and stated that this would represent an unacceptable change in the protocol of discussions and be detrimental to the medical laboratory service.

The Institute ensured that members were made aware of the intentions of the DHSS, which resulted in a flood of correspondence and much debate in branch and regional meetings. Such was the level of reaction that questions were raised in the House of Commons concerning the effect of these proposals on patient care in the NHS.

After two further meetings with the DHSS, the Institute reached an agreement that was issued in July 1976 in Health Notice (76,130) entitled *Training of Medical Laboratory Technicians, Study Arrangements for the Special Examination of the Institute of Medical Laboratory Sciences*, which included provision of 20 days' release for course attendance. Clearly, this was insufficient for an approved course but was a great improvement on existing regulations. Similar provisions were introduced in Scotland and Wales, as was an agreement for release to the course operating at Ulster College in Northern Ireland.

***

The Institute issued a number of policy statements during the 1970s on staffing and management issues and in 1976 was invited to give evidence to the Royal Commission on the National Health Service. The Institute highlighted the lack of progress towards achieving an integrated staffing structure for scientific staff and criticised the outdated and unrealistic arrangements for management of laboratories set out in two DHSS publications, HSC (IS) 16, *Organisation of Scientific and Technical Services,* and in June 1978, (STS) Z 132/23, *Scientific and Technical Services in the NHS*.

These comments attracted hostile reactions from some pathologists who believed that the views were directed at their role. It is quite clear that they felt threatened, which was far from the intention, nonetheless the Institute tried to quell any animosity by publishing a statement entitled *Pathologists and Ourselves*. This sought to clarify the roles of the medical laboratory scientist and the pathologist; on clinical issues there was no dubiety but there were areas of disagreement regarding laboratory management.

Throughout these times the Institute continued cordial relations with The Royal College of Pathologists (RCPath) through the regular meetings of the Standing Joint Committee of the IMLS and the RCPath. Even when there were differing views expressed by the Institute, effective dialogue was always maintained.

Relationships with The Association of Clinical Biochemists and The Association of Clinical Pathologists (ACP) were less harmonious during this time. It appeared that the source of much of the sniping at the Institute and the profession was from elements within the ACP, particularly from those expressing their views that were appearing in the British Medical Journal (BMJ) at that time.

An erudite analysis of this professional conflict was contained in a report prepared by Professor Roger Dyson of Keele University, entitled *The Management of Pathology Laboratories* (1977). Professor Dyson was commissioned by the ACP to prepare the document, although some parts of the report were probably overlooked if they did not suit a particular stance. Another article by Professor Dyson appeared in the BMJ in December 1978, entitled *Who Manages Pathology Laboratories?*, which also gives a good insight into the same issues.

***

In 1978 an acrimonious dispute developed in Scotland regarding management arrangements in the Fife Area Laboratory, when the Fife Health Board sought to reduce the role of the Principal Medical Laboratory Scientific Officer. The situation arose in relation to the interpretation of management roles in the laboratory following a Parliamentary statement that appeared to endorse the view that hospital laboratories should be managed by medical consultants or non-medical scientists of equivalent standing. A bitter trades union dispute ensued, the principal protagonists being the Association of Scientific, Technical and Managerial Staff (ASTMS) and the British Medical Association (BMA).

The matter was made worse by the ACP, when it published its own version of model job descriptions for senior medical laboratory scientific officer posts. This was regarded with contempt as both professional interference by one body to another and undermining the Whitley Council arrangements set out for determining conditions of service.

As a result, an independent three-man inquiry into management arrangements in the Fife Area Laboratory was established in 1979, following a proposal from the Scottish Home and Health Department (SHHD). The Institute was approached by the SHHD to make a nomination to serve on the inquiry, albeit in a personal capacity. The findings of this inquiry were reported in confidence to the Fife Health Board. The Institute tried on numerous occasions to seek release of the report, without success.

Initially, the Institute believed it faced a dilemma when asked by the SHHD for a nomination to the inquiry. It believed that had it refused then the SHHD would have chosen someone to support its position, rather than nominate an individual who would be independent of the SHHD and exercise good knowledge of management issues. Clearly, the Institute made the right choice with its nomination of Mr Graham Smart to the inquiry, but he had to maintain confidentiality in not disclosing the details of the report.

***

The beginning of the 1980s was heralded by a strike of steelworkers, which was settled with the agreement of a 17% pay award; however, there were to be no further bonanzas of this sort. The policy of the Thatcher government was to face down any further wage demands backed with the threat of strikes with direct confrontation, which resulted ultimately in the infamous miners' strike of 1984–85. Despite this gloomy backdrop, progress and innovation in other areas was evident. Probably the most notable in everyday life was the availability of affordable home or personal computer.

The Institute continued to develop its education and qualifications programmes but was constantly finding itself involved with attempts to resolve long-running NHS issues, including the integration of scientific staff and management issues related to the Fife dispute, which had not been settled despite five years of bitter wrangling.

In January 1982, Mr Graham Smart began his tenure as President of the Institute. In the 10 years since he was first elected to Council, Graham Smart had been a very active and visible figure in Institute affairs. He had visited many branches and was keenly sought as a speaker; a role in which he excelled. It would not be an exaggeration to suggest that the election of Graham Smart heralded the expectation of a strong figure who would stand up for the Institute and its members in a contentious environment. This was clearly evident when he addressed a meeting of the North region in Middlesbrough on 6 November 1981, and spoke on 'The Profession Under Attack'.

As a role model, he exemplified the opportunities open to those with the resolve and ability to achieve personal advancement while enhancing the profession. He supported educational opportunities at undergraduate and postgraduate level so that medical laboratory scientists could exercise their full potential and in doing so enhance the standing of the profession.

Graham Smart was born in 1938 in the Welsh valleys. He began his career at Cardiff Royal Infirmary in 1956 and went on to pass the Intermediate examination in 1959 and achieved Fellowship in 1963. He then moved to a senior post at the Royal Berkshire Hospital in Reading before returning to Cardiff in 1965 on securing a chief's post in the Research Unit at the Dental School. He had a keen interest in management and recognised the importance of the development of general management principles that were being introduced in the public service environment at that time. This led him to study for a Diploma in Management Studies, achieving the award in 1974. It is likely that he was the first member of the profession to gain this qualification. He continued his studies and in 1976 obtained a BA in Philosophy and Social Sciences. In 1977 Graham Smart was appointed Principal MLSO at Southampton General Hospital, where he worked until his retirement.

Following his first election as a Council member in 1972, Graham was soon elected to the Executive Committee where he served until 1992. He was appointed Vice President in 1995 and Chairman of the International Association of Medical Laboratory Technology (IAMLT) in 1996. On his election as President some Council members expected that his strong personality would lead to conflict with the General Secretary, John Fawcett. This was not the case as both men had been acquainted long enough to have gained mutual respect and understanding, and their partnership at the helm of the Institute has to be one of the strongest in its history, and much credit must be accorded them in this respect.

Graham was a member of many education committees representing the Institute across the United Kingdom and in Ireland. In 1980 he also carried out a three-week sponsored lecture tour of South Africa in conjunction with the Congress of the International Association of Medical Laboratory Technologists. Even after his retirement from Council, he was surprised to find that he was still recorded as a member of committees he thought he had long given up.

***

In 1982 the Institute reported that its costs had been subjected to an annual inflation rate of 11% and had shown an operational loss in the previous year. As a result there was a substantial increase in subscription rates – the first for four years – bring the annual rate for Fellows to £28, Associates £23 and Students £12. A comparison with other medical societies showed that the Institute's rates remained the lowest. Despite this rise, the overall membership showed a small increase to reach 16,953. Previously, when membership fees were increased in 1975 and 1978, there had been a decline in overall membership.

In respect of industrial disputes in which Institute members found themselves during the preceding period, and the requirement for the Institute to publish a public declaration of its stance, Council felt it necessary to produce a new code of conduct, to be adopted by all members. An earlier version had been published in 1957. The Council adopted the new code of professional conduct at its meeting held in March 1982 (Appendix).

***

Throughout the history of the Institute, there has been almost continuous debate among the membership regarding an explicit role for the Institute in the negotiation of terms and conditions of employment for its members. This is despite regular explanations of the Memorandum of Association that clearly states that the Institute's terms of reference preclude it from this role. The attitudes of Department of Health officials and its advisors towards medical laboratory staff in the NHS during the late 1970s and 1980s hardened belief that the Institute should be fully involved in negotiations on behalf of its members. Among the implications for the Institute in adopting a trades union role would have been its loss of charitable status, with dire financial consequences, and result in an inevitable increase in membership fees.

During the early 1980s this issue featured increasingly in correspondence to *The Gazette* and in resolutions being put forward from branches and regions. As a result, in 1983, Council acceded to these proposals and established a working party to examine the possibility of adopting a trades union role. The original report of the working party was rejected on the grounds that it did not adhere to its terms of reference.

A further report resulted in Council rejecting the proposal on five counts: i) existing unions could not have been expected to agree to surrender seats on relevant Whitley Council committees to permit a new union to be represented, and in becoming a union the Institute would have lost its consultative status; ii) it had been evident from informal discussions after the 1983 Annual General Meeting and correspondence during the year that many members working in the NHS would not have wanted the Institute to take on a trades union role; iii) the Institute's assets would need to be transferred to another charitable institution and the resources raised to sustain a new union would probably have been insufficient to support the full compass of union activity; iv) skilled union staff and a regional network of offices would have been required, at great expense; and v) the existing reputation of the Institute in the scientific and academic spheres, which had ensured that its professional advice was respected, would have been undermined.

Following discussion after the Annual General Meeting at the 1983 Triennial Conference in Stirling, it was emphasised that a substantial majority of members would have to support a change in role for the Institute for that decision to be seen as authoritative. At the Council meeting held in December 1983 it was formally agreed that the Institute should not seek to form a trades union.

***

During 1982 the Institute celebrated the centenary of the birth of its founder, Albert Norman. A dinner was held in the Hall of Trinity College, Cambridge, on 16 July. Those attending included Mr Harry Hobson, one of the original signatories with Albert Norman of the Memorandum of Association in 1942, and Mr Sidney Laws, a member since 1919, who actively campaigned for the formation of the Institute as a limited company.

In 1912, at the age of 29, Albert Norman founded the PBLAA that became the Institute in 1942. He died in 1964 but his wife, Florence, survived him and her attendance at the event was greatly appreciated. The principal guests at the dinner were Sir David and Lady Price. Sir David was Vice President of the Parliamentary and Scientific Committee, to which the Institute belonged. In his response to the President's address, Sir David remarked on the appropriateness of the venue in respect of Albert Norman's early place of work and the great changes that had taken place since his birth.

***

The death occurred on 4 February 1983 of Mr John Hatcher. A former Council member, John will best be remembered for his regular articles in *The Gazette*, beginning in 1971, featuring pioneers of medical science and historic instruments. John Hatcher had also encouraged the collection of such instruments that became the official collection of the Institute, amounting to over 1300 items. At the Triennial Conference at Sheffield in 1974, discussions took place to form a group that would seek to record the practice and instrumentation of past eras. The Historical Section was formed, with W H Valentine the first chairman and Dr A D Farr and G C Pascoe (who had taken over the chair by 1978), with John Hatcher its first secretary. A G W Webb succeeded Hatcher as secretary and carried out a large amount of the work involved in cataloguing the instrument collection.

In 1982, at a meeting of the Joint Working Party on Historical Instruments of the Institute and The Royal College of Pathologists, it was agreed that the collection of instruments would be transferred to the Science Museum for safe storage and preservation, a process completed in 1984. Members of the Historical Section regularly presented exhibits of historic instruments and notable discoveries at Triennial conferences, beginning in 1974, and have continued at every subsequent Institute Congress event.

In 2007 the Historical Section changed its name and status to become the History Committee, with defined objectives and a responsibility to Council, and it continues to have a good working relationship with the Science Museum.

***

Council had been debating a change in the membership structure of the Institute during the four years to 1983. Paramount in any changes was the preservation of the rights of current Fellows and Associates. The final proposals were published in February 1983. In explaining the position of the existing structure, it was pointed out that the Institute's structure was unusual in that it was the inverse of that operated by many similar societies. It was therefore understandable that many organisations had difficulty in recognising the status of Institute members in relation to those of other learned societies.

It is not usual for the highest qualification of a professional body to be gained relatively early in a career and also to be held by a large proportion of the membership, which was the situation prevailing for Institute members. A further example was the class of Associate, which was the second highest level of Institute corporate membership, but usually regarded as a non-corporate class of membership by most other bodies. The structure also required that graduate entrants to membership be in the class of Student in the first instance, which was clearly not an encouragement to recruitment.

Under the new proposals, all current Fellows would remain in that class and continue to use the post-nominal letters FIMLS. Associates would also remain as before and use AIMLS until they qualified for a higher class of membership. The proposed structure would have four classes of non-corporate membership: Affiliate, Student, Associate and Licentiate, with two classes of corporate membership, Member and Fellow. Arrangements would also be kept in place for members to be granted honours comparable with the existing titles of Vice President, Honorary Fellow, Life Member and Member in Retirement. Extensive consultation with the membership was undertaken through the branch and region structure, with correspondence recording opinions in *The Gazette* with responses and developments from Council.

Council agreed to complete the proposals in 1985 and put them forward as Special Resolutions at the 1986 Annual General Meeting in Southampton, at the Triennial Conference. Although there was a majority vote in favour of the resolution (For 471, Against 296), it was not sufficient to enable the three-fourths majority required to create a change to the Articles of Association. Council was therefore unable to proceed with plans for the changes. It took until 2008 to implement a new structure with redefined entry to, and classes of, Institute membership.

***

The Council meeting held in December 1983 was notable for the appointment of the President Elect. It was recorded that there had been two nominations, Mr A J Barrow and Mr R G Fewell, the latter having been the Institute Treasurer since 1979. Robert George Fewell was announced as the President Elect at the 1983 Annual General Meeting in Stirling, to serve from January 1984.

At the same Council meeting, Arthur John Barrow was elected as the

Treasurer, to serve from January 1984, to succeed Mr Fewell. This decision resulted in a constitutional inconsistency. Mr Barrow was the South West region Council member at that time and the Articles of Association state that he could not remain in this office and become Treasurer simultaneously. The Articles did, however, allow a member to be coopted to fill the regional role (coopted members had to be confirmed at the next round of Council elections) but it was felt that such an appointment could influence the voting process at the next Council elections in June 1984. Nevertheless, it was decided to invite Mr Barrow to continue in his office as South West region member for the next few months until Council elections took place.

Mr Russell T Allison was elected to serve as South West region Council member at that election, an appointment that was to have great significance for the development of the Institute in years to come.

The Gazette reached a milestone in April 1984 with the publication of the 400th issue. When first published in January 1951, *The Gazette* comprised six pages with 10 advertisements and a circulation of 4550 copies; however, by 1984 the Institute's monthly publication had a distribution of 18,000 and brought news, informative articles, classified advertisements and educational courses to all classes of member, as well as through libraries to many other interested parties.

***

The presidential term of Mr Robert (Bob) Fewell commenced in January 1985 and may have been seen as the return of a figure linked with the past. Bob Fewell commenced his career in 1940 at The London Hospital in Whitechapel and spent his whole working life, apart from a two-year period serving in the Royal Navy, in the same establishment. He was the Principal Medical Laboratory Scientific Officer from 1961 until his retirement.

Bob had a long association with education through organising courses and teaching Institute students on the Intermediate and Final courses in haematology. He was appointed a Final Examiner in 1958 and served on the Examining body until 1971.

Elected as a national member of Council in 1968 and appointed to the

Executive Committee in 1971, he was re-elected annually until his election as Treasurer. He also served on many other committees, notably the Finance Committee from 1969, serving as its chairman for 10 years from 1973, during which time he was appointed Treasurer.

During his first year of office, he presided over a unique Annual General Meeting of the Institute. On 8 June 1985, the AGM was held in The Court Hotel, Killiney Bay, near Bray, 10 miles south of Dublin. The first and only occasion to date on which the AGM of the Institute had been held outside of the United Kingdom. The meeting was memorable for the venue and wonderful hospitality of the Dublin branch but also for two special events: first, Mr S G Laws MBE FIMLS, was presented with Life Membership, having been a member since 1919 and influential in the change from the PBLAA to the Institute; and second, as a result of the recent Council elections, the outcome of which marked the end of the Council membership of Mr T S Lansley OBE FIMLS, who had served for 27 years since 1958 and had been Chairman from 1967 until 1969. In a tribute, Bob Fewell said that there had been few matters of importance that Tom Lansley had not been personally involved during his membership of Council.

The 1985 Council elections also saw Mr E J Cloke gain the highest number of votes when he was re-elected as a national member. The support for Jim Cloke may well have been due to his chairmanship of the newly convened Medical Laboratory Scientific Officers National Advisory Group (not an Institute body), which closely monitored the appointment to Principal posts and pathology management issues in the NHS. There was a consistent view, held by many members, that despite clear decisions to the contrary, the Institute should play a greater role in these issues.

In discussions following the AGM, Jim Cloke spoke during a debate on medical laboratory scientists' perceptions of themselves. Following the reported comments in *The Gazette* by the General Secretary when addressing the Fife Health Board, in which he wrote: "The role of the scientist was to produce data and that the role of the medically qualified consultant was to interpret such data". Jim Cloke observed that the need for hospital pathologists to interpret data was rapidly declining and consequently so was their consultative role. This evolutionary process was becoming a handicap to the scientific profession as pathologists were in many cases trying to take on managerial and administrative responsibilities to supplement their diminishing role. The profession had pioneered the qualification in medical laboratory management, which was held by many senior medical laboratory scientists.

The public image of medical laboratory science as a profession was not identifiable at this time. In correspondence to *The Gazette* in September 1985 from R L Ward JP FIMLS, entitled 'As Others See Us', he summarised the issues confronting the profession and the Institute. "The need for us as a profession to 'go out and sell ourselves' is not only necessary; it is vital for our survival. The divisive government policies which state that we do not 'deal with patients' and are therefore not to be mentioned in the same (negotiating) breath as nurses and doctors, deals us a severe blow. It relegates medical laboratory scientists to a professional backwater, which no amount of graduate recruitment or postgraduate degrees will overcome. Any body of workers, professional or not, that has no industrial strength, or alternatively does not have widespread public sympathy, can expect nothing. It is unrealistic to think of medical laboratory scientists as being any longer industrially strong. There is no public sympathy and, by definition, no support where there is no public awareness. Even within hospitals, few other groups could accurately describe medical laboratory scientists' professional duties and responsibilities, let alone educational requirements and long training programmes."

Mr Ward implored Council to "Get to grips immediately with the issue of public relations and to do so with enthusiasm. Regrettably, power politics are the only method of achieving results and modern publicity techniques need to be employed expertly. Justice, I am sorry to say, has little chance of success".

***

Opinions as expressed by Mr Ward sat uncomfortably with Council, on two counts: first, that adopting a confrontational stance was alien to the

Institute's policy; and second, the Institute was inexperienced in the practice of public relations and therefore did not venture into unknown territory.

However, in 1986, following recommendations from the Publicity and Services Committee, Council decided to engage a professional public relations company to investigate the needs of the Institute and draw up recommendations and agreed initial funding of £6000 for the research. The brief, which was sent to those companies bidding for the commission, included the following: i) to note the Institute's constitutional objectives and how to improve its operates; and ii) to indicate what could be done to improve its 'public relations' and what the cost would be. The target audience should encompass not only the public but also ministers and departments of government, educational bodies, medical and other health service professions and professional bodies. It should also target existing and potential future members of the Institute.

A number of specific objectives to be considered were included in the brief, namely: publicising and utilising the scientific and managerial roles, activities and achievements of medical laboratory scientists; improving relations with members and promoting concord and unity among them; attracting and retaining the membership of those eligible to join; promoting professional awareness among members; and utilising the *IMLS Gazette* and other resources as effectively as possible.

The Institute and its members were experiencing increasing levels of attack on their professional position, both as an organisation and as individuals. The provocation was mainly coming from government in respect of its refusal to recognise the status of medical laboratory scientists carrying out the diagnostic analysis so integral to the delivery of healthcare, and the reality that many senior members of the profession were performing effectively in their managerial positions.

The Institute did attempt to address some of these issues through the establishment of management courses and examinations around the United Kingdom and continued communication with the Secretary of State for Social Security, often to correct erroneous statements referring to the profession.

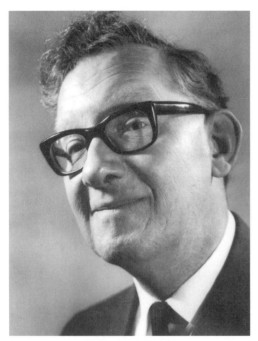

Walter H Finch

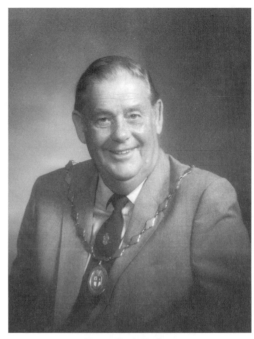

Francis J Baker

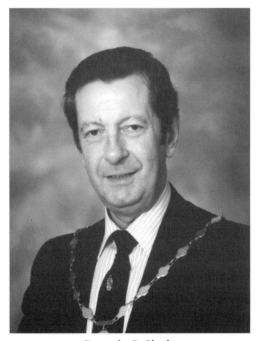

Dennis B Slade

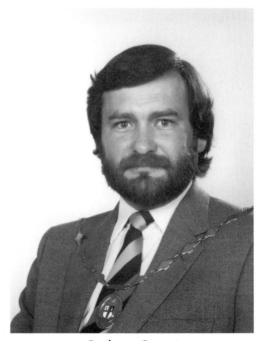

Graham Smart

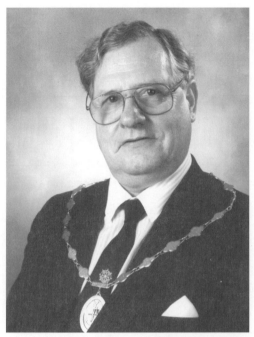

Robert G Fewell

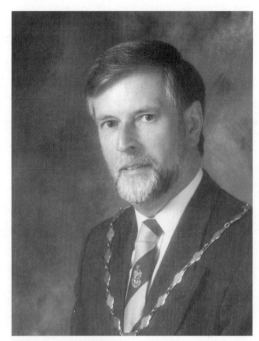

E James Cloke

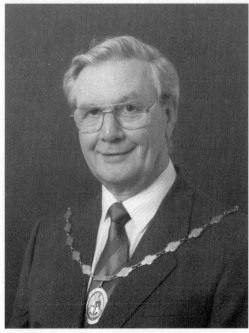

Arthur J Barrow

***

In 1986, Council was moved to publish a restatement of the objectives of the Institute in the prevailing environment. The Memorandum of Association, which stated the original objects for which the Institute was established, namely, to promote the study and to promote the development of medical laboratory sciences. Whatever the Institute does must therefore be directed to improving the efficiency of the medical laboratory service in all its manifestations within the public and private sectors. Detailed objectives designed to address the efficiency of the medical laboratory service were specified: i) promoting research and development ii) improving standards of professional education and laboratory training, and enhancing efficiency and cost-effectiveness through structural changes, particularly the integration of medical laboratory scientists in the NHS; iii) organisational changes, particularly good management of the service; and iv) practical changes, such as those resulting from the evaluation of laboratory buildings, equipment and tests.

Council felt that these statements represented the interests of the members in addition to enhancing the scope of the profession as a whole.

***

The 18th Triennial Conference of the Institute of Medical Laboratory Sciences was officially opened on Sunday 17 August 1986 by Professor A P M Lockwood, Chairman of the Biological Council and Professor of Oceanography at the University of Southampton, where the event was held. The traditional Albert Norman Memorial Lecture was given by Professor R R A Coombs, best known for giving his name to the antiglobulin test used in transfusion science.

As remains customary, Council held a meeting on the preceding day, at which Mr E J Cloke was elected President Elect to serve until Mr R G Fewell completed his three-year term as President at the end of 1987.

Mr Cloke was appointed to Council in 1976 and had been a member of the Executive Committee since 1984 and was also chairman of the Medical Laboratory Management Committee. It is unlikely that he could have envisaged the changes at the Institute that would ensue during the next four years of his office.

The 1986 annual general meeting held on Monday 18 August had been publicised regularly as a potential milestone in the history of the Institute when the special resolution to change the membership structure of the Institute was put to the vote. It had taken nearly seven years of debate and preparation to reach this stage. In the event, the resolution failed as it did not receive the three-fourths majority required. This was viewed with great disappointment by Council and it immediately began a review of the details of the resolution, with the objective of representing them at the next AGM, to be held in London in 1987. There was much further debate and Council members visited many branches to explain the changes to the original resolution that had been incorporated as a result of suggestions from members.

The revised special resolution was presented at the 1987 AGM held in the Edward Lewis Lecture Theatre at the Middlesex Hospital in London.

The President Elect, Mr E J Cloke, introduced the special resolution by reiterating that important differences had evolved in the Institute's structure compared with other scientific and educational bodies. He said that members should see the changes as a benefit to the profession and not as any individual loss of status.

After lengthy discussion at the meeting, the vote resulted in another failure of the special resolution, the extent of the defeat being greater than that of the previous year (For 552, Against 788), the majority of the votes against being cast by proxy.

***

During 1987, several very public issues occupied the attention of Council and the Institute. An article published in *The Daily Telegraph* on 14 July 1987 reported that the British Society for Clinical Cytology (BSCC) had alleged "poor or non-existent training of laboratory technicians", contributing to 2000 avoidable cervical cancer deaths a year. Many complaints about the article were received by the Institute, and members also wrote directly to the newspaper, strongly refuting the content of the report. This followed the disclosure that a large number of cervical smears had been incorrectly reported in Liverpool.

Earlier in April 1987, senior Institute representatives had met with the Minister of Health, Antony Newton, and had discussed the recruitment and training of staff in cytology and the introduction of a quality control programme. Clearly, there was a need to unify the criteria of entry into cytology with that of the other disciplines in medical laboratory science.

The source of the original disclosure was the widely reported misdiagnosis of 911 false-negative cervical cytology smears by a consultant pathologist, identified as Dr Kathleen Lodge. When the mistakes first came to light, several false and unsubstantiated accusations were made about the medical laboratory staff working at the Women's Hospital in Liverpool. A report published by Liverpool Health Authority, entitled *Internal Review into the Laboratories at the Women's Hospital, Liverpool,* stated that there was "no logical explanation for Dr Lodge's mistakes" and it also criticised another pathologist, Dr Percy Jones, for not responding to the situation and not taking action when the medical laboratory scientific officers in the cytology laboratory had expressed their concerns to him.

The report praised the medical laboratory scientific officers and said that "in the absence of their initiative, this problem would have remained undisclosed". When this report was released, the Institute realised there would be much publicity. In order that the responsible work of the medical laboratory scientists would not be eclipsed by misreporting, as so often seen in the past, the Institute undertook an intensive press relations campaign to explain the role of medical laboratory scientists and promote its objective for a national system of quality control in cytology laboratories.

Council appointed Mr Russell Allison to join Mrs Jan Gauntlett, representing the BSCC, and also head of the pilot study into quality assurance in cervical cytology, to act as Institute spokespersons on the day of the report's publication. It also contacted major newspapers and television stations, resulting in the appearance of reports in *The Times* and *The Daily Telegraph*. A further press release was issued from the Registered Office following the announcement by health minister Edwina Currie that double checking of all cervical cytology smears would be undertaken.

This episode highlighted the need for specialist skills in the practice of public relations; an issue that Council had been considering over the previous year. The cytology situation resulted in a 'baptism of fire' for the Institute because the subject was so politically and publicly sensitive. The membership also realised the need to be prepared to undertake public relations in a professional way, and an increasing number of articles and meeting reports on the subject began to appear in *The Gazette* at this time.

***

Soon after the first reports on acquired immune deficiency syndrome (AIDS) appeared, attempts to understand the clinical aetiology of the condition had become a major interest, and this led to a change in practice in many areas of medical laboratory science, including an increase in workload due to the soaring demand for human immunodeficiency virus (HIV) tests.

At a meeting of Institute representatives with the Minister of Health, Antony Newton, the subject of AIDS was discussed. The Institute had two nominated experts on the Advisory Committee for Dangerous Pathogens, and they had been involved in the publication of guidelines on the handling of material suspected of containing HIV. It was pointed out that medical laboratory scientists were frequently depicted by the media carrying out HIV testing, and, while there was an understanding of the risks involved for these staff members, there also needed to be recognition of their role in the allocation of resources to meet the increases in workload, including the impact on staffing and consumables costs.

Chapter 13

Progress by Degrees, Diplomas and Certificates

In the late 1940s, when the NHS was launched, a university education was out of the reach of many who aspired to obtain a degree. After a somewhat protracted gestation period, The Open University (OU) accepted its first students in 1971 – all 25,000 of them – and the so-called 'University of the Air' was finally up and running. Breaking the link between exclusivity and excellence, the OU flourished and grew in tandem with the digital age. Passage of the Further and Higher Education Act 1992 *allowed all polytechnics to become universities, and 38 took up the offer of metamorphosis immediately, nearly doubling the number of universities in the UK.*

As has already been seen, the first graduates became members in 1936 and from then on a steady trickle joined the profession. Many senior members of the profession were at best ambivalent and at worst antagonistic to graduates. It is said that this opposition arose from the attitude of a small number of graduates who believed that their qualifications were superior to Institute qualifications. However, some may well have been due to inverted snobbery by senior members of the profession who did not think much of the practical ability of graduates.

By 1949 the number of graduates entering the profession had risen and it was agreed that exemption from the Final examination would be granted to holders of a science degree or an Associateship of the Royal Institute of Chemistry, with at least one year's experience in an approved laboratory. Entrants with these qualifications were then permitted to qualify for Fellowship by thesis or dissertation after a further three years' experience. This was changed in 1956 and graduates with one year's experience could sit a Final examination. At the same time, holders of an HNC in chemistry, with five years' experience in a chemical pathology laboratory, could gain exemption from the written and practical parts of the Final examination in chemical pathology. However, they could only obtain Fellowship by thesis or dissertation in chemical pathology.

Further changes were made in 1960 when overseas graduates were able to sit a Final after two years' training. In the mid-1960s, holders of higher degrees from British universities were given exemption from the Final examination for Associateship. The opposition to graduates lessened in time and in 1967 Council announced plans to develop higher qualifications of degree status.

**

Two changes were introduced in 1968. The first was that UK science graduates would be made Associates without having to take any further examinations, and the second allowed holders of higher degrees with appropriate experience and Institute membership could, at the discretion of Council, be elected to Fellowship. During the same year, a committee of educationalists, members of the profession and Institute representatives presented draft proposals for a qualification of degree status. This became the ill-fated Diploma in Medical Technology. It was suggested that IMLT members who had at least seven years' experience and who had an HNC in Medical Laboratory Subjects could enrol on a course for the diploma. The course would comprise a Part I of 300 hours part-time study, plus a Part II of 800 hours part-time study. Although Regional Hospital Boards agreed to release technicians for the course, the DHSS, without informing the Institute, instructed the Regions to postpone action on requests for the course. As the IMLT had kept the Health Ministry fully informed of the development and the course was co-sponsored by the Department of Education, this was a massive shock. Council reacted strongly and the DHSS eventually agreed to the release of 15 students per year, nationally, but of the three courses originally proposed only Sir John Cass College was able to run one. The first award was made in 1972 and the last intake was in 1975, after which it was no longer offered.

Although it was short-lived, the qualification achieved the aim of the IMLT to produce a qualification of degree status. It was recognised as the equivalent of a good Honours degree in 1973 by the Burnham Further Education Committee, in 1975 the DHSS and Scottish Health Department recognised it as appropriate for appointment, under Whitley Council PTA regulations, as a scientific officer, and in 1976 the RCPath accepted it as a suitable qualification for entry to the MRCPath examination under its Honours degree regulations.

***

Towards the end of the 1960s the increasing importance of the management role of senior laboratory staff was recognised. However, there was no specific training or qualification available for this role. In view of this, a working party was established to advise on the establishment of a course and examination. It produced recommendations and a study guide which were approved by Council in September 1969. It was for a two-year course, with one study weekend per year, open to Fellows of the Institute (it was possible for Associates to be admitted to a course at the discretion of Council). Colleges were invited to submit schemes for the course for approval by the Institute. The examination was set by the Institute in consultation with the colleges, and successful candidates were awarded the Certificate in Medical Laboratory Management (CMLM). Following a review in 1979 the qualification was further developed and became the Diploma in Medical Laboratory Management (DMLM).

The course was popular but suffered from two drawbacks. First, there was no provision for time off to attend the courses – health service management viewed the qualification as an 'optional extra' and not essential. Second, it was viewed by those outside laboratories as too specific and not transferable to other health service management roles. Also, more general management training and courses including MBAs were becoming available in the NHS, and, as they were widely recognised, they were preferred by many senior staff. Taking account of this, the Institute had discussions with the Institute of Management with a view to developing a Diploma in Managing Biomedical Sciences. It was also hoped that there would be an element of reciprocity with the qualifications of the Institute of Health Service Management. However, after considering the proposals, it was argued that hospital management was changing rapidly and that the Institute could not dictate biomedical science content for a management programme. The proposed qualification was not introduced. The last DMLM examination, except for re-sits, was held in 1994.

***

By 1974 about 10% of those joining the Institute and about 20% recruited as medical laboratory technicians were graduates (not all of those employed as technicians in NHS pathology laboratories joined the Institute). At about this time polytechnics and universities began to explore the possibility of offering degrees the content of which could broadly be described as Honours degrees in biomedical science. Initially, these were through the inclusion of appropriate modules in already established science degrees, although later specialist degrees became available.

As in early 1968, the University of Aston had proposed an Honours

Degree in Medical Laboratory Technology but the Institute had declined to support it, partly because the Institute's own scheme (Diploma) was under consideration, and partly because it awaited the report of the Zuckerman Committee. In 1974, Portsmouth Polytechnic, utilising a modular science degree that had been adapted from an external London degree, introduced a major option in medical laboratory sciences, validated by the CNAA. The programme comprised modules in cell biology and chemistry together with a major physiology component, and was approved by the CPSM and IMLT for state registration and Associateship, respectively, following one year's training in an approved laboratory. The title was Joint Honours Programme in Physiology and Medical Laboratory Sciences, and the first students graduated in 1977.

The University of Bradford, utilising its basic philosophy of sandwich degrees, announced a B Tech. in Medical Sciences in 1975. The third year of the course was spent working and training in an appropriate, approved laboratory. For CPSM training purposes, the sandwich year counted for state registration for the UK health services. The first graduates completed the course in 1979.

Several other polytechnics and universities expressed interest in these new undergraduate topics and entered the field. As a result, the Institute began to advise them and accredit their degree programmes. By the mid-1980s there were at least 10 specialised MLS degrees in the UK and more were planned.

The two pathways, HNC or degree, for CPSM registration and Associateship, continued in parallel until the early 1990s. The 1992 Triennial Conference was, in more than one way, very influential on the development of the IMLT. It was agreed at the AGM held during the Conference that, from the autumn of 1993, students should enrol on relevant Honours degree courses rather than HNC/D courses. However, steps were taken to ensure that anyone who commenced an HNC/D course in 1992 and did not pass would be given sufficient time to re-sit examinations as necessary.

***

The Institute had anticipated that full-time education would not be appropriate or possible for everyone. It believed that there would be a demand for part-time courses and took advice from experts in MLS education. A plan was developed for part-time vocational degrees and the feasibility of this was discussed widely. There was some concern that the courses would be too long, but it was recognised that credit could be given for appropriate laboratory-based education and training, and if this was taken into account then the courses could be shortened. Progress was rapid and four part-time degrees were accredited by October 1992 (Sheffield Hallam, Liverpool John Moores, Westminster and NESCOT). Alternative models were developed at the University of Ulster. The West Midlands RHA sponsored students at Wolverhampton University and arranged vacation and sandwich placements for them.

At the beginning of the 1990s many healthcare-related professional bodies took the view that they should move to an all-graduate entry. The CPSM took a similar view and from 27 September 1993 required all new registrants to have an appropriate degree. The involvement of the Institute in the examination system was further reduced when in1994 it was announced that the last examination for Fellowship would take place in 1997. With the ending of Scheme 'O' in 1993 and the DMLM examination in 1994, for the first time since 1921 the Institute no longer set or marked its own examinations (except for those members examined by thesis). As a result many in the profession again questioned the need to remain members of the Institute, or indeed for its continued existence.

***

From 1995, an applicant for Associateship of the Institute needed to hold an approved or accredited Honours degree. The main involvement of the IBMS in formal education became the accreditation and approval of BSc and MSc degree courses. It achieved this by working closely with the Heads of University Centres of Biomedical Science (HUCBMS), which was formed in 1993 in association with the Institute. Fortunately, some members of Council and senior officers of the Institute realised that attitudes and events in the wider world would have major implications for the membership, particularly those employed in the NHS.

In the early 1990s, high-profile legal cases highlighted problems with laboratory quality and service provision for the NHS Cervical Screening Programme (NHSCSP). Partly as a result of this a shortage of pathologists willing to participate in the programme became apparent. In some departments this gap was filled by the ad-hoc appointment of clinical scientists, but at that time there was no statutory regulation of, or formal qualification for, these posts. As a result, the IBMS and RCPath were asked by the NHSCSP to devise a training and qualification scheme for these posts. The Institute had already introduced the Certificate of Competence in Cervical Cytology in 1989; in 1995 this was replaced by the NHSCSP's Certificate in Cervical Cytology Screening. In 1998, the IBMS examination in Interpretive and Diagnostic Cytology was introduced, but was replaced in 2001 by the examination of the Conjoint Board (IBMS and RCPath). This then became the necessary qualification for appointment as an Advanced Biomedical Scientist Practitioner in Cervical Cytology (this qualification is now known as the Advanced Specialist Diploma in Cervical Cytology).

***

Two further changes, after the millennium, had major impacts on the role of the IBMS as a provider of qualifications and certificates. These developments greatly enhanced its responsibilities and influence.

The first of these was replacement of the CPSM by the Health Professionals Council (HPC) on 9 July 2003. While the new body was responsible for the regulation of the professions and the registration of practitioners, many of the duties of the CPSM were no longer the responsibility of the HPC. The IBMS took over the issuing of logbooks (later to become the Certificate of Competence Registration Portfolio), the approval of laboratories, the issuing of certificates of competence for registration, and the assessment of qualifications.

The second was *Agenda for Change* (the title given by the Department of Health to a major overhaul of the NHS grading and salary structure) which was linked to the Knowledge and Skills Framework (KSF; a competence framework designed to support personal development and career progression within the NHS) and National Occupational Standards.

The IBMS took the opportunity to develop a series of certificates, diplomas and examinations that could be used as evidence of attainment, as well as routes to Membership and Fellowship of the Institute (from January 2006 the previous grades of Member, Associate and Fellow became Licentiate, Member and Fellow, respectively). These were, in many ways, significantly different from the type of examination set previously by the Institute. Originally, Institute qualifications were by examination, with some continuous assessment and project work introduced in later years. The new system relied much more on the use of portfolios and structured laboratory-based training.

The Specialist Diploma, a discipline-specific qualification, is designed to facilitate post-registration training as well as complement the theoretical knowledge obtained by MSc. It is obtained by a laboratory-based training programme equivalent to two years' practice and final assessment of a training portfolio. The Higher Specialist Diploma was launched in 2003, initially as an examination to test candidates' competence to practise at a high level within their chosen biomedical science discipline. The candidates' abilities are assessed by a combination of a portfolio, case studies, essays and examination. These qualifications are complemented by Certificate of Expert Practice examinations, which are designed to demonstrate knowledge and skills in specific areas such as electron microscopy, quality management and mycology. Diploma of Expert Practice examinations are aimed at those with an MSc and cover clinical transfusion, diabetes, histological dissection and immunocytochemistry. Fellowship by Thesis has become the Diploma of Higher Specialist Practice, and ophthalmic pathology and specimen dissection have been added to cervical cytology as subjects covered by the Advanced Specialist Diploma.

With this wide range of awards, the IBMS re-established itself as a vital provider of qualifications for those working in and around pathology. Further recognition of the Institute's role in maintaining the high standard of education, training and continued competence of its members came in 2004 when The Science Council awarded the IBMS Licensed Member Body status. This allowed it to confer Chartered Scientist (CSci) designation on appropriately qualified and experienced members.

***

During the 1980s there was increasing political and public distrust of many professions. Self-regulation and the apparent lack of systems to ensure that individual practitioners kept their knowledge and skills up to date came under scrutiny. As far as Medical Laboratory Technicians were concerned, state registration covered the first concern but there was nothing, other than professional pride, to ensure that they kept up to date. Indeed, there were people working in pathology who, once qualified, neither attended a meeting nor read a journal, and made no effort to maintain their knowledge. There was, however, growing recognition that all professionals need to update their knowledge and expertise regularly. The Institute had, since its inception, provided a range of educational activities designed to keep members up to date, but there was no formal scheme for post-qualification Continuing Education and Training (CET) or Continuing Professional Development (CPD).

In September 1989, Council set out objectives for a CPD scheme, invited proposals for CET short courses, and asked Russ Allison to chair a committee to review any proposals. A Leader in the November issue of *The Gazette*, written by Russ Allison, explained the rationale behind the scheme and the plans for its development. It was hoped that the objectives could initially be met through short courses, symposia and formally structured meetings. It was intended that additional activities such as structured home reading, projects, distance-learning and sessions at large meetings would become a formal part of CPD and that a scheme of credit accumulation would be adopted. The first courses were advertised in March 1990.

Major changes were made to the CPD programme in 1992 when, on 1 May, the IMLS CPD Diploma was introduced. This was a comprehensive scheme that allowed all members to "have their personal updating and professional commitment formally recognised". Participants were required to register for the scheme and pay a fee of £20, which kept the member on the

CPD register for five years. Following registration, they received an information pack and an activity record card. Activities were divided into two classes – educational and professional – and organisers of events were required to apply to the Institute to have them accredited. Each activity was allotted a set number of credits, depending on length and type. A diploma was awarded when a total of 25 credits (60% of which needed to be in the educational category) had been obtained. Retrospective credits were also available for all recognised activities undertaken since the scheme's launch in 1989.

The scheme was kept under review and 'fine tuned' from time to time. However, many participants found it difficult to attend meetings and courses. The government and employers were not always supportive and study leave and financial support was not always available. In an attempt to address these difficulties, two new activities were introduced in 1995 – the Structured Reading Programme and Journal Based Learning. Further minor modifications were made and a review in 2002 – the 10th anniversary of the CPD Diploma – led to the introduction of a new portfolio, a new credit system and the addition of reflective learning.

By this time, what had been an optional scheme started to become essential. The NHS was subject increasingly to inspection and scrutiny. Practitioners in all professions needed to produce evidence of CPD and CTE, and participation in the IBMS scheme fulfilled this requirement. When the Health Professions Council replaced CPSM as the statutory regulatory body in 2002, it was made clear that CPD would become a requirement of continuing registration. In July 2006, the HPC required all health professionals on its register to undertake CPD as a legal requirement, and the IBMS produced CPD profiles that would accord with this requirement.

Chapter 14

Biomedical Science Congress

A New Beginning

Early in the 1990s a tearful Margaret Thatcher was seen to depart from 10 Downing Street, a home she occupied and dominated since first passing through the famous black portal in 1979.
Use of the internet expanded, and the Hubble telescope encountered early problems; a dockyard electrician and a lawyer previously incarcerated for 25 years became presidents of Poland and South Africa, respectively; and the launch of a new motor car in Birmingham had an unforeseen effect on a new scientific gathering.

The IMLS Council published a Development Plan during 1991 which was to have far-reaching consequences for the Institute and its Triennial Conference. As a consequence, a Meetings Focus Group, comprising members of the discipline-specific scientific advisory committees, chaired by Mr Tony Harding, was formed early in 1992, to make recommendations to Council. Of the areas it was asked to consider, two were most apposite, given the difficulties to come, and were to review critically the Triennial Conference and consider alternative models, and to increase cooperation with commercial conference and course organisers. The group was also asked to give consideration to the cutting-edge scientific content of future meetings and to explore the possibility of sessions based on major themes, rather than specific disciplines.

The group reported to Council in May 1992 and made nine important recommendations, those relevant to the conference were: i) that 1992 be the last Triennial Conference, ii) in 1994 the venue should satisfy the higher expectations of delegates, speakers and exhibitors, iii) a Scientific Programme Committee should be formed, iv) the conference should remain multidisciplinary in format, v) guidance on ensuring a corporate image was needed, and vi) the views of members and Company Members should be sought. In addition, the group produced a checklist against which potential conference venues could be judged

**

During 1992 the Institute formed the Company Membership Scheme and a Company Members Liaison Group, which comprised Company Members and Institute officers. It held its first meeting in April 1992, which was perhaps fortuitous as it provided a forum for the discussion of the problems experienced during the Liverpool Triennial. Keeping potential exhibitors informed of developments and taking heed of their views meant that, when the decision to completely revamp the Conference was taken, support and the assistance of the Company Members was assured.

After considerable deliberation, and a report from the Conference Committee, Council decided to look for professional conference organisers to undertake the administrative arrangements in the name of the Institute and to find a venue more suited to the needs of a prestigious conference. The only aspect of the organisation retained by the Institute was the design and organisation of the scientific programme. Of four companies interviewed, Reed Exhibitions was selected as the most suitable. With its help a number of potential venues were investigated, including Brighton, Harrogate and Birmingham International Conference Centre (ICC).

At the end of May 1992 a draft business plan for the next major Institute conference recommended Birmingham as the most suitable venue. Not only was it a modern, prestigious venue, with all the necessary facilities in close proximity under one roof, it was the venue favoured by potential exhibitors. A booking was made for September 1995 but the ICC management reneged on the booking, preferring instead to hold a major launch of a new car – Birmingham at that time was a major centre for automobile manufacture. To compensate, the ICC offered the Institute a considerable reduction in hire cost, and it was agreed to hold the meeting at the end of October.

***

The above notwithstanding, other problems needed to be overcome, the first of which was what to call the meeting. A new meeting needed a new name, one that distinguished it from the accumulated problems of the Triennial series. Several names were considered and eventually 'Biomedical Science Congress of the Institute of Biomedical Science' – in 1994 the Institute of Medical Laboratory Sciences became the Institute of Biomedical Science – was chosen as the most appropriate. While this title describes the event, it is generally referred to as the 'Biomedical Science Congress', or just 'Congress'. A further departure from the past was the plan to hold Congress every two years.

The two elements of Congress, the Scientific Programme and the Exhibition, were treated as two separate financial ventures, with any profit or loss being shared equally between the Institute and Reed Exhibitions (later Step Exhibitions). Although Reed Exhibitions was being hired to run the administration of the Congress, it remained the Institute's meeting, with all letters, literature, communications, publicity and marketing under the

Institute heading, and no public reference to Reed Exhibitions.

As previous conferences had been based in universities, inexpensive student rooms were available for delegates, and could be booked as part of the conference fee. Birmingham Convention and Visitor Bureau (BCVB) provided an accommodation booking service for delegates to Congress but individuals were to be responsible for booking their own accommodation. There was concern that this would deter junior members, so, as an alternative to potentially expensive hotel rooms, accommodation at Aston University was made available, and transport between the university and the ICC was arranged. However, this proved far from ideal as the service was relatively limited, and many delegates found it difficult to return 'home', change and return for social events. This arrangement was discontinued in 2001.

***

The first session of the new Congress event could perhaps be viewed as a fringe meeting, as it was held in a hotel the evening prior to the official opening. It was a joint session between clinical chemistry, haematology and management, entitled 'A Pathology Service – Back to the Future?'. The official opening was on Tuesday 31 October 1995. The IBMS President, David Browning, noted in his welcome that it was not only the first new-style meeting, but also the first since the Institute changed its name, the first in Birmingham and the first in an integrated conference centre.

The scientific programme was more ambitious and complex than had previously been attempted, with over 210 presentations, papers, workshops, discussion sessions and quizzes, held in 15 lecture halls or rooms, presided over by 47 different chairmen, plus three days of poster sessions covering nine disciplines or topics. Not only were there parallel sessions but some disciplines used several meeting rooms simultaneously. On Wednesday there was a plenary session, held in conjunction with the Association of Clinical Pathologists, entitled 'The Health of the Nation'. After the opening section, at which Professor Sir Colin Berry gave the Albert Norman Memorial Lecture on 'Risks, Health and the Environment', three parallel sessions on cancer, epidemiology and life-style illness were held.

As the organisers wished to ensure that Congress was perceived as a major scientific meeting, any activities viewed by them as peripheral to this aim were not included. The Annual General Meeting was probably not missed by the majority of members, but the lack of a social programme was mourned, as the various tournaments, visits and sightseeing tours were no longer part of the meeting. Many of the participants who completed the feedback questionnaires remarked that "everyone was scattered all over Birmingham and there was no chance of meeting old friends". As an original object of the conference, going back to the first in 1924, was networking, so this was something that needed addressing before the next Congress. Nevertheless, some activities were organised, including a Council and Friends Cabaret Evening in aid of the IBMS-nominated charity, the National Kidney Foundation, with an opportunity to meet 'Sidney the Kidney'. A total of £1532 was raised during the Congress for this charity.

***

After the problems encountered with the Liverpool Triennial in 1992, there were fears that space in the exhibition would be hard to fill, but these concerns were unfounded. All the space was taken within weeks of it being made available. Over 120 stands were taken and several companies were unable to book space. In addition, 32 companies provided generous sponsorship for the scientific programme. The feedback from the delegates and exhibitors was generally very good and it was felt that, although there were lessons to be learned, the new format and arrangements had proved to be a great success, and it was decided to hold the next Congress in 1997 at the same venue.

In 1997, Congress was reduced to three days. It started on the Tuesday with a plenary session on gene therapy, followed by the official opening ceremony, and the scientific programme commenced in the afternoon and ran to the Thursday afternoon. Bearing in mind the feedback on the first Congress, some social events were arranged. These included a Welcome Evening, the President's Reception and a Company Members Evening, plus 'Happy Hour' on the Tuesday and Wednesday evenings in the exhibition hall.

The second Congress also saw the introduction of the Cybercafé. Although other venues were investigated, it was decided to use the ICC again for the 1999 Congress, and what followed built on the successful pattern of the two previous events.

One advantage that the planners had was continuity. To a great extent, each Triennial was a new venture, as the experience and knowledge acquired by a branch when organising the event was not available to those of another branch organising the next Triennial. Formation of a Congress Committee, which included the professional organisers, representatives of the Company Members, members of the scientific advisory committees and Council members resulted in the introduction of some stability to the organisational process. The same personnel were able to plan and review Congress and build a body of knowledge and experience that could be used to develop and improve Congress.

***

By 2001 the pattern for Congress was well established and, although the number of delegates increased each year, more attended on the second and third days than on the first. Analysis showed that the plenary session was not popular, and changes were made to the 2003 programme in an attempt to overcome this problem. Registration began on Sunday afternoon and the scientific programme commenced on Monday with eight parallel sessions covering all the major disciplines. The formal opening and plenary session was moved to the afternoon and concentrated on professional and political matters relevant to biomedical scientists, both inside and outside the NHS.

The emphasis on 'issues of the day' in the Monday afternoon plenary session proved to be a great success. The number of delegates attending the first day rose from under 700 in 2001 to nearly 1200 in 2003, and has remained proportionally the same in subsequent events. Issues ranging from the developments in education, the *Agenda for Change* programme, career development, the Carter reviews of NHS pathology, and pathology networks all attracted a large audience and lively debate.

Each Congress has built on the success of its predecessor and introduced new features. Participation of the National Association of Phlebotomists in 2003 and the Association of Anatomical Pathology Technology in 2005 recognised the close links the IBMS and pathology has with these groups. In 2005, delegates were given the chance to learn basic life support skills, have a health check, and take up opportunities to meet members of Council and the Executive to discuss professional issues on a one-to-one basis. In addition, seminars on pathology in primary care were organised for those faced with the prospect of involvement in point-of-care testing.

***

Although Congress is no longer a branch-organised event, the role of the local IBMS members remains crucial to its success. A team of IBMS members drawn from the Birmingham area has been organised by John Foster, each tasked with a role designed to make Congress run more efficiently. They prepare the conference bags, man a help desk, look after the speakers and chairmen, staff the media suite, liaise with ICC staff and generally assist the smooth running of Congress.

An unexpected consequence of the switch from a university-based meeting to one held at the ICC was the apparent change in the demeanour of the delegates. This has been remarked upon by members who were regular attendees of the Triennial. In their view the attitude, standard of dress and behaviour of delegates is much more 'professional' than previously was the case. Whether this is due to their surroundings, accommodation or justifiable pride in belonging to a professional body able to hold a meeting in such a prestigious venue remains unclear.

Chapter 15

The Institute as an Expert Witness

In the 1979 film Monty Python's Life of Brian, *Reg asks: "All right... all right... but apart from better sanitation and medicine and education and irrigation and public health and roads and a freshwater system and baths and public order... what have the Romans done for us?" However, it would be quite easy to substitute this with the question: "What has the Institute done for me?"*

Much of what the Institute does and has done – examinations, education, conferences, advertising job vacancies – is very visible, but perhaps much more is unseen and less tangible; even for that which is visible there is, inevitably, considerable background work not exposed to the light of the public gaze. It is, depending on one's view, an iceberg or a swan!

The Institute has always taken a broad view about what constitutes members' interests. The direct issues of knowledge, education, qualifications and career advancement have to some extent been covered elsewhere in these pages. However, there have been many other issues on which it has been consulted, expressed a view, or initiated discussion that have had great influence on the profession in the UK and abroad. The Institute has become the 'Expert Witness' for its profession and for many aspects of laboratory practice. Many other bodies have views on various aspects of the profession, but only the Institute, together with the appropriate trades unions, is truly qualified to represent biomedical scientists.

Officers and senior members of the PBLAA were consulted by some employers, sat on a joint committee with the PathSoc and had lobbied the War Office about the role of Assistants during the First World War; however, as a result the developments in the organisation of healthcare and education in the second half of the 1940s, the views of the newly-formed IMLT were more often sought.

In 1944, as well as continuing to sit on the joint committee with the PathSoc, representatives of the Institute sat on the Joint Services Committee, sat on or met with the Joint Services Pathological Committee, the Joint Committee on Salaries and Wages (Hospital Staffs), representatives of the Ministry of Health and the Association of Scientific Workers. As a result, the Ministry of Health agreed that the Institute should be recognised as a tutorial and qualifying body for medical laboratory technical personnel and that the Institute would be regarded by the Minister of Health as the appropriate body for consultation on matters of major importance.

The Joint Services Pathological Committee, which had representatives from the Army, Navy and Air Force pathology services, the Association of Clinical Pathologists and the Medical Research Council, agreed unanimously that training of technicians in the three services should conform to Institute standards and that the technicians trained in all three services should be encouraged to sit the Intermediate examination. In 1944, the Association of Scientific Workers took the view that it was desirable for all laboratory technicians to hold the qualifications of the Institute.

When National Service was introduced – from 1946 until the beginning of the 1960s, men aged 18 were required to undertake two years' military service – the Institute was able to persuade the authorities to allow student technicians to defer starting their military service until they had reached the age of 21 years. This gave them enough time to study for and to sit the Intermediate examination.

The Joint Committee on Salaries and Wages (Hospital Staffs) invited the Institute to discuss national scales of salaries. It was hoped that the committee would also consider the advisability of adopting Institute qualifications for admission and advancement, and thereby secure a means of controlling the professional status of laboratory technicians. This was not implemented at first but was accepted eventually by the Whitley Council. The Institute never secured seats on the NHS Whitley Council, but three members attended in an advisory capacity and were accepted by both sides as independent arbitrators. Even in this role, they were often the subject of criticism, and blame, for decisions on remuneration that were outside their control.

***

There is no doubt that a laboratory scientist with Institute qualifications was recognised, as Albert Norman put it, as "the genuine article". The massive expansion of pathology in the 1960s, not only in the number of samples submitted but also the range and complexity of investigations offered, plus the introduction of automation, put greater pressure on laboratories to ensure that their results were accurate and reproducible. While the Institute introduced quality assurance schemes of its own (eg dye approval), it was in collaboration and consultation with other professional bodies and with the Department of Health that it had a major influence on the development and introduction of laboratory quality assurance and accreditation.

Many laboratory professionals viewed participation in external quality assessment as a slight both on their integrity and skill. Nevertheless, many laboratories recognised potential problems and developed informal studies into inter- and intra-laboratory comparability of results. These led to awareness of the need for improved laboratory quality control and the introduction in 1969 of National Quality Control schemes for clinical chemistry and haematology. Under the auspices of the Advisory Committee on Analytical Laboratory Standards and the Joint Working Group on Quality Assurance, these schemes evolved into the UK National External Quality Assessment Scheme (UK NEQAS). The Institute has always played a major role nominating senior members to these bodies and committees to represent opinions and knowledge of the profession in these matters.

During the 1980s there was increasing public and political pressure on professions to provide evidence of the reliability and quality. For the individual, this led to the introduction of continuing professional development (CPD) and continuing professional education (CPE), but this did not test the reliability of the laboratory service as a whole. Consequently, in early 1989 the Institute wrote to the Department of Health (DH) about accreditation of laboratories. Although internal quality control (IQC) and external quality assessment (EQA) schemes had been running for almost 20 years, participation remained voluntary. The IMLS believed that they should be mandatory and as a consequence some form of laboratory accreditation should be introduced, overseen by an independent licensing authority. In its reply, the DH pointed out that it had raised this issue in its consultation note on Management and Staffing of Pathology Services and that it was awaiting responses. It also indicated that it would follow the RCPath pilot accreditation scheme proposals with interest and expressed the view that it was sure that the Institute would have a major contribution to the debates on these topics.

After conducting pilot inspections in 1990, the RCPath invited the IMLS and other interested bodies to join a steering committee. Institute observers were present for the second round of pilot visits, after which further modifications were made to the scheme and it was recognised that both pathologists and biomedical scientists should inspect laboratories jointly, and this became standard practice. The Institute nominated senior members of the profession as inspectors, and, in 1991, Cheryl Blair, an Institute Fellow, was appointed as the project manager (in the following year Cheryl became Executive Manager) and further pilot inspections were undertaken with IMLS-appointed inspectors.

Following further modifications to the process, a company to administer the new scheme for accreditation of diagnostic laboratories in the UK was registered on 6 January 1992, and Clinical Pathology Accreditation (UK) was born. The Institute and the RCPath were the major shareholders – three and four shares, respectively – and a further 12 shares divided between the Institute of Health Service Management, Association of Clinical Pathologists, Association of Clinical Biochemists and the Independent Heath Service Association. In April 2009 all the shares were purchased by the United Kingdom Accreditation Service (UKAS); however, CPA continues to function under the UKAS umbrella, with senior Fellows of the Institute acting both as professional full-time and peer-group discipline assessors.

Changes in technology during the 1980s gave rise to tests and equipment that could be used outside the formal laboratory setting to provide information for the diagnosis or monitoring of treatment – so-called near-patient testing (NPT) or point-of-care testing (POCT). If used by individuals who had been well trained, using properly maintained equipment and reagents that had been correctly stored, these methods gave valuable information, but this was not always the case. An added concern was the increased use of these tests outside a healthcare setting.

Tests for cholesterol became available in shopping arcades and other places and there was usually no control over the validity of accuracy of the results. There was no requirement for those involved in NPT, in or outside healthcare, to take part in EQA or similar quality control systems. Concerns about the quality of NPT and the safety of high-street testing – sometimes dubbed 'pavement pathology' – were raised by the IMLS in 1992. Its campaign aroused the interest of the press, and Institute Chief Executive Alan Potter was quoted in *The Guardian* and a Council member was interviewed on television. These concerns led to the Institute issuing guidelines on POCT in

1992, which were updated in 2004. The Institute worked closely with the DH, RCPath, CPA and other relevant bodies, including health service management and the nursing profession, to raise awareness of the potential hazards of POCT. Eventually, it became a requirement that health service management should ensure that POCT undertaken within their purview be performed using equipment selected with the help of pathology personnel, with properly trained staff and a quality and safety management system in place. These arrangements are under the control and scrutiny of a qualified POCT manager, who is usually a biomedical scientist with appropriate Institute qualifications. This has helped to ensure that investigations undertaken outside the confines of pathology are subject to the same stringent controls as those performed within the laboratory, and to a great extent have eliminated the risk of incorrect results endangering the safety and well-being of patients.

*****

The Institute has sought to maintain the quality of training and appointments within the NHS by using the expertise and experience of its senior members, thus ensuring that employers enjoyed the benefits of Albert Norman's "genuine article". Over the years, the Institute has provided advice on suitable external assessors for appointment panels, model job descriptions, members of grading appeals panels, lists of individuals suitable for appointment as CPA assessors, Council for Professions Supplementary to Medicine (CPSM) inspectors, portfolio examiners, and in many other cases where a professional and independent opinion was needed.

The Institute has always sought to lead the profession on matters of probity and quality; this was generally achieved through publication of articles in *The Gazette* and presentations at specific meetings. While this kept members informed, disseminating this information to the wider community was more difficult. During the late 1990s, it began to publish policy statements, professional guidance and quality standards as leaflets for wider dissemination. Among these were a Code of conduct and Code of practice for biomedical science laboratories; Guidance on BSc degree course accreditation; Near-patient testing; Patient sample and request form identification criteria;

Staffing; Giving results over the telephone; Error logging; and Workload in UK clinical diagnostic laboratories. Over the next decade the advice in these leaflets was kept under review, revised, re-issued and added to as new developments emerged that affected the profession and the practice of pathology. Not all advice was issued in isolation, however, as on a number of issues the Institute worked closely with other relevant bodies. For example, in 2007, it worked in collaboration with the RCPath on the issue of guidelines on the handling of medico-legal specimens and evidence.

Guidance and opinion was also disseminated through *The Gazette* and during the revision of the *Guide to good professional practice for biomedical scientists* the focus group produced comments and advice on items, perceived at the time to be crisis issues, such as extended-day working, combined laboratories, on-call, skill mix and 'hot labs'.

***

The Institute has an important history of representation on a wide range of advisory bodies and committees. Its nominees have contributed to many highly significant reports and publications, and continue to do so. A glance at *The Gazette* or an Annual Report shows that it has been represented on bodies as diverse as the Dangerous Pathogens Advisory Group, the various committees of the British Standards Institute, the European Committee in Clinical Laboratory Standards, and, in the context of the Institute's responsibility to promote and maintain standards, advice was given to many NHS trusts and units undertaking local reviews of pathology services.

The *Annual Report 2000* illustrates the range of consultation and liaison that took place, with meetings with the DH, RCPath, National Advisory Group for Scientists and Technicians in the NHS, The Pathology Alliance, Allied Professions Forum, CPSM and CPA. In addition, it was invited to express views on subjects as diverse as Healthcare scientists – a case for change; Modernising regulation – the new Health Professions Council; A health service for all the talents: developing the NHS; Supporting learning for PAMs in Scotland; Routes to state registration for biomedical scientists (Wales); and a draft report on a national service specification for haemophilia.

A survey showed that Institute members were an important source of information on diagnostic testing. As a consequence, the British In Vitro Diagnostics Association proposed collaboration with the Institute and others in promoting the use of diagnostics as a means of prevention as well as cure, and the Institute joined the campaign in an advisory capacity.

***

As well as providing the more obvious professional services to its members, it has introduced a number of services of a more material nature. At a time when members experienced problems in obtaining copies of scientific papers, either due to the lack of access to a journal or a photocopier, the Institute provided a photocopying service. It has, on occasion, negotiated various other benefits for members including, at one time or another, preferential rates for car and household insurance; discounts for electrical goods, tailoring and sports equipment; group subscription to a car breakdown service; reduced premiums for unit trust investment; a credit card; a mortgage service; and even special arrangements with the Royal Overseas League to allow members access to the facilities of this residential West End club.

Corporate clothing has also featured from time to time, with the Institute selling items such as scarves, ties, badges (lapel, car and blazer), sweaters and polo shirts all bearing the Institute Coat of Arms or logo. In 1976, for the first time, members were provided with a diary.

At the beginning of 1991 the Institute took this a stage further and contracted with Bishopscourt Financial Services for a package of personal financial and insurance services for members. This not only added value to membership but also acted as a recruitment and retention inducement as well as a source of income generation for the Institute. Without doubt, however, the most important service to members was the introduction in 1991 of Professional Indemnity Insurance, the cost of which was included in the annual membership subscription fee. It provided professional and monetary protection in the event of legal action being taken against an individual for malpractice and/or public liability in cases arising out of the performance of their professional duties.

***

The Institute can be said to have entered the digital age in 1980. The accounts for that year show an entry for the 'Hire purchase of a computer – £55,500'. The equipment was used for internal administration, records and the administration of examinations. However, it was not until much later that the Institute harnessed the power of the internet. It launched its first website just before Congress in 1997; however, it took a further two years before a recognisable email address (mail@ibms.org) was integrated with the website.

The stated aims of the new website were to describe the aims and work of the IBMS, give details of Congress, summarise the CPD scheme, outline the Institute's activity in science and professional education, provide information on publications and enrolment. A members' discussion forum was added in 1998. Generally well received by the membership, the website was enhanced by facilities to enable online Congress booking in 1999, and links to region and branch networks arrived in 2000; however, by 2004 it was starting to show its age and was revamped and relaunched. This updated site won the *Laboratory News* Best Scientific Resource Website in 2004. The *eNewsletter* was launched in 2001 to keep members in touch with news, local events and other items of interest.

The ability for members to access lectures, speeches and reports on Congress was added in 2003, and online CPD records arrived in 2010. A further major update and relaunch was undertaken in 2010, and in the same year digital communication went beyond the web into Facebook and Twitter.

Chapter 16

Nineties and the Noughties

An Aura of Excitement

Early in 1991, in Scandinavia, Harald V became King of Norway, while in the sands of an area once known as Mesopotamia, Operation Desert Storm was successful in freeing the small Emirate of Kuwait from Iraqi occupation. A decade later, on a day in September 2001, an aura of incredulity descended on the world following the attacks on the twin towers of the World Trade Center in New York and on the Pentagon outside Washington DC. Another decade later and a prince and his new princess emerged from the Great West Door of Westminster Abbey, watched by billions of people around the world.

The end of the 1980s and the early 1990s was an era of great change and upheaval for both the Institute and the profession. This was a period when the NHS generally, and pathology specifically, came under considerable scrutiny, resulting in several publications that proposed or introduced major changes. Key among these were the Management Advisory Service (MAS) *Review of Pathology Services* (Mowbray Report), the Department of Health (DH) circular EL(89) P/171 *Management and Staffing of Pathology Services*, the government White Paper *Working for Patients, Working Paper 10*, the Whitley Council PTB Committee A agreement on restructuring the NHS pathology grades, and the consultation paper on a possible integrated structure for non-medical staff in NHS pathology laboratories. The introduction of the 'internal market' to the NHS caused further insecurity. Laboratories that had previously collaborated found themselves in competition, not just with each other but also with private sector laboratories, some of which had been developed specifically to take work away from the NHS. Many laboratories were amalgamated or closed.

For those working in NHS pathology departments the uncertainty that these developments engendered caused a great deal of anxiety. Many members, perhaps not entirely unfairly, were critical of the Institute. There was a feeling that the Institute was impotent and unable to influence events. However, many of the areas of concern were matters for the trades unions and not a professional body. The Institute even re-examined the possibility of becoming a trades union, but it was realised that this was impracticable as it would have led to loss of Charitable Body status, which would have had a severe impact on the finances of the Institute. It also took the view that to become a trades union would have an adverse effect on its responsibility for the promotion, development and recognition of the profession and the setting and maintenance of professional standards. There was also no possibility of the IMLS gaining seats on the Whitley Council. So, yet again, it was decided not to pursue a trades union role but to remain a professional body and learned society.

Changes in the education system, together with those to the grading structure in NHS laboratories, and the qualifications needed for senior posts, led many members to question the need for the Institute and the value of membership. Many members did resign from the Institute and the number of new recruits fell, leading to a large reduction in membership.

Some of the developments that took place during this period are dealt with in more detail elsewhere, including CPD, accreditation, professional indemnity, membership services, company membership, the move towards an all-graduate profession, as well as the creation of the Institute's Conference Unit and Education Department in 1992, the latter having a pivotal in the formation of the Heads of University Centres of Biomedical Science (HUCBMS) group. Some were new initiatives while others resulted from a great deal of soul-searching analysis of the role of the Institute.

***

In February 1988, John Fawcett, from 1962 the Deputy General Secretary and from 1970 the General Secretary, retired. John, who became an Institute Fellow in 1952, was awarded the Sims Woodhead Medal in recognition of his long and distinguished service to medical laboratory science and the Institute. His contribution to the Institute was further recognised in 1989 when he was elected a Vice President.

He was replaced by the first person to have the formal title of Chief Executive, Dr Hilary Lodge, who took up his duties on 1 March 1988. Although from outside the profession, on paper he was well qualified for the post, being a chartered secretary with an MSc in business administration and a PhD for research at the London Business School. Prior to his appointment, he had worked for Vickers, Courtaulds, English China Clays, in Independent Television, and at the Institute of Energy. He was a business-orientated manager, not an academic or scientist. As an outsider, he was perhaps able to take a more objective view than those who had been intimately involved in the running of the Institute.

His first impressions, which were published in *The Gazette* in July 1988, were that there was a great deal of uncertainty about the role of the Institute. He accepted that all institutions tended to grow rather haphazardly over time and become preoccupied with keeping the system going, with little time to take stock. To address this he suggested that the small working party, which had been invited by the Executive Committee to review the committee structure, should first devote its efforts to a review of the Institute's aims and objectives. Council subsequently identified four strategic objectives: to develop a continuing education programme, improve and sustain communications, promote the Institute, and identify and develop commercial activities. During 1988 the committee structure and their terms of reference was reviewed but it took a further two years to implement these changes, when the number of Council committees was reduced from nine to six. The scientific advisory committee structure was retained as were the advisory committees for Ireland, Northern Ireland, Scotland and Wales.

Hilary Lodge also felt that as the vast majority of members were employed in the NHS the Institute was in effect "industry captive" and stated that "when the NHS took a hammering, the IMLS appears to take a hammering. The Institute is not seen as a separate entity from the NHS but appears to be part of it". Most people would disagree with his view about the Institute appearing to be a part of the NHS, but he was right when he said that when attacks were made on the NHS at that time, the Institute's members attacked the professional body "for not doing enough". Morale in NHS pathology was very low, engendered by uncertainty, poor salaries and a feeling that the status of the profession was under attack.

Although Hilary Lodge clearly identified areas which the Institute needed to address to improve its relevance, effectiveness and image, his appointment proved less successful than had been hoped. His unauthorised attempts to obtain a Royal Charter brought him into conflict with Council, and his contract was terminated in September 1989.

Miss Heather Tate took over as Acting Chief Executive until the appointment of Alan Potter in June 1990. At the time of his appointment, Alan was Assistant Unit General Manager at St Margaret's Hospital, Swindon, where previously he had been Principal MLSO. Therefore, he was well acquainted with the Institute and the problems of the profession, and had wider experience of the NHS and how it operated at a senior management level; knowledge and experience that was to prove invaluable to the Institute during the turbulence of the next few years.

***

Mr Jim Cloke, who became President at the beginning of 1988, was acutely aware of the dissatisfaction of the membership and the view that the IMLS was out of touch, information not obtained solely from IMLS activists. At that time, each NHS Region had a series of committees which advised their Regional Scientific Officer on matters relevant to their service. Each Region had an MLSO Advisory Committee and representatives of each of these committees sat on the National MLSO Advisory Group. Jim Cloke had been chairman of this group for several years and also had good contacts with the trades unions, so he was aware of the feeling across the country and the depth to which morale had fallen.

As a first step to improve communications with the membership, plans were made to ensure that every Institute branch was visited by a Council member at least once a year and to invite observers from branches to Council meetings. This was followed, towards the end of Jim Cloke's presidency, with a series of President's Workshops for branch and region officers. These were held in London, Birmingham and Newcastle upon Tyne at the end of 1990, with one for Irish officers in early 1991. Their purpose was to obtain input and direction from the grass roots into the development of Institute policies and services. The topics which arose at these workshops were then raised at a briefing and training workshop for branch secretaries. The subjects covered local recruitment, local needs, local promotion and the *Local Officers' Guide*. The headings and comments from the syndicates at one workshop gave a good indication of the low morale apparent even in active members. They were very critical of the Institute, commenting that the "IMLS sits on the fence", it is "perceived to have lost control of education", has "no sense of identity", and asked "Is there a continued need for Fellowship?" Syndicate headings included 'despondence', 'moribund', 'failing', and 'demoralised'. However, it was not all bad news as there were many good examples of local and national initiatives which helped to enhance public awareness of the profession.

These workshops were followed by a Council workshop. The first task was to attempt to answer the question "What is Council for?". This may well have been the first time such a question had been asked by Council of Council. The answers were perhaps obvious but served to focus Council's thinking about how the Institute functioned and should develop.

Four focus groups – Income Generation, Organisational Structure, Publications, and Relationships with Other Bodies – were established to develop the future strategy. These deliberations, together with recommendations from the Chief Executive, resulted in the production of the IMLS Development Plan, a short version of which was published in *The Gazette* in April 1992. Unfortunately, the authors have been unable to obtain a copy of the final printed report. Nevertheless, the short version sets out the objectives of the five-year business plan clearly. Business planning and business plans were then a new concept for the NHS. The introduction to the plan states: "The Institute ought to cooperate with others in achieving its ends, and it ought to be proactive and not always be exclusively identified with the National Health Service. It should seek to enhance its corporate image and the collective image of its members, and to improve the effectiveness of its Council, committees and office staff. The plan is a statement of strategy and policy that will permit the Institute, in a rapidly changing environment, to maintain or increase membership and to prosper".

It was a plan that would radically alter the way the Institute functioned and it influenced its development for many years. The areas to be considered were identified under nine major headings: Organisational Structure, Scientific Programme, Relationships with Other Bodies, Publications, Income Generation, Education, Membership, Public Relations and Council Activity. Each section examined the issues to be addressed and, while options were put forward, few if any hard and fast proposals were made.

Improved communication with the membership was seen as essential to ensure that individuals felt involved in the decisions made by Council. The implications of Working Paper 10, which allow the involvement of employers in the evolution of professional education, as well as the moves towards European standardisation, were recognised as issues to which the Institute would need to be equipped to respond. Stronger links with industry and the expansion of membership were seen as important for income generation. The former was already bearing fruit through the Company Members scheme. The plan recognised that the principal direction of the education strategy had already been decided; however, it realised that the Institute needed to be proactive in its dealings with employers and those who would provide the degree courses.

The importance of a high-profile scientific programme was also recognised. Perhaps key to the future development of the scientific programme were the scientific advisory committees (SACs), but communication between the SACs needed improving. A review of the role of the SACs and their terms of reference was proposed, together with a hope that they would link closely with the CPD scheme. A review of the Institute's conference was already underway but it was felt that a high scientific profile was essential, irrespective of the final format.

***

The task of bringing the plan to fruition was the responsibility of Council and its committees, together with a special working group and input from the branches. It also needed changes at the Registered office in Queen Anne Street and support from its staff. However, it was a working plan, the report on which concluded by saying: "It is important (for it) to remain dynamic, and the plan should be updated on an annual basis". This plan laid a firm foundation for the changes that occurred over the next few years.

In June 1992 the Organisational Structure Focus Group, which had been given the task of reviewing the region and branch structure and its terms of reference, presented its report to Council. It proposed a change to the division of the UK and Ireland, from seven regions with 48 branches to 12 regions with 47 branches, and that each region should be represented by a member of Council. It also considered the suggestion that there should be 'specialist' Council members. It concluded that these specialists were not required as advice was available from the Education committee and SACs. After consultation with branch and region representatives, modifications were made to the proposed structure, reducing it to 11 regions with 48 branches.

Perhaps the first sign of the change in approach was the new Institute logo. It was announced in *The Gazette* in June 1990 and first used therein the following month. In his letter to the membership announcing this new logo, Jim Cloke said: "The IMLS has long been established as the voice of medical laboratory scientists. With the changing pace and demands of healthcare and its sciences, however, the need now is not only to consolidate that position but to sound the voice more loudly. This is vital not only to maintain credibility but also to ensure a clear, dynamic image that matches new demands and competitive elements". The design, by Hartnell Design Associates, fused the DNA double helix with the symbol of the staff and snake of Aesculapius. The four lines symbolised the four main divisions of medical laboratory science, and the colour exploited the established marking image for science and medicine, with an upward spiral to illustrate the universal and continual search for ever-higher standards in academic qualifications. The logo was intended to underline the professionalism of IMLS members and to reinforce the Institute's public image. The initial cost for the design and development was just under £20,000. Not everyone was happy with the introduction of a logo, feeling that the Institute's Coat of Arms was, and should be, the public symbol of the Institute.

Quite a lot of attention in the Development Plan was given to relationships with other bodies, which were seen as fundamental to the activity of the Institute. There was a realisation that, with the devolution of decision-making within the NHS, it required the ability to exert influence at local, regional and DH level in the future. Beyond this there was the importance of relationships with bodies active in the same fields as the Institute. Regular meetings with the RCPath, ACP and ACB were envisaged, together with closer contact with single specialty groups (ie NAC, BSCC, BBTS, BSHI) as well as with the other professions covered by the PSM Act and the CPSM. In the Annual Report 1992, Council reported that liaison with other bodies had improved. Subsequent annual reports contained accounts of meetings and joint initiatives with a wide range of professional and other appropriate bodies.

As part of its ongoing review, Council agreed in 1993 that there should be a new mission statement setting out the Institute's aims: "To promote and develop biomedical science and its practitioners, to establish and maintain professional standards, and to be the influential professional body in biomedical science". Although written in more expansive terms typical of the 'management speak' of the time, the sentiment remained true to one of the founding principles of the PBLAA: "To assist in the general advancement of its members".

***

The new grading structure for NHS pathology staff was announced at the end of 1988. This reduced the number of grades from seven to five and introduced the new grade of Medical Laboratory Assistant (MLA); a non-career grade for support staff. Implementation of the new structure took considerable time and the uncertainty of individuals about their future position and grade engendered much anxiety within the profession.

The new structure potentially had severe implications for the Institute as senior grades (MLSO2 and above) were no longer required to hold Fellowship of the Institute. The Institute's response to this was to issue a statement saying that in its view it was "important that senior members of the profession retain the requirement for Fellowship when appointing appropriate staff to posts in their laboratories. Any departure from this will jeopardise the status of our profession and the ability of our medical laboratories to serve properly the interests of patients". This view was supported by the DH and in reality most employers continued to require the qualification for promotion to supervisory grades. However, many members took the view that membership of the Institute offered them no advantage. New entrants to the profession did not need to join in order to obtain qualifications, and established members in senior posts did not need to retain their membership once promoted. As a result, between 1988 and 1990, total membership fell by nearly 20%, with the number of Associates and Fellows falling by almost 18%.

There was concern that the new post of Medical Laboratory Assistant (MLA) could further undermine the status and role of qualified staff. In

December 1988, Council asked the Regulations Committee to consider what provision could be made in the Institute's membership structure for the admission, if appropriate, of cytoscreeners and MLAs. After some consideration, it was eventually decided that there was no place for these staff groups within the Institute. It did, however, work closely with the ACB, ACP and RCPath to produce a joint view on the role and duties of MLAs. This made it quite clear that this grade was not part of the career pathway, and that any MLA wishing to become a trainee MLSO could only do so in open competition with other applicants. With these and other relevant bodies, it agreed a competence logbook to be used to record the training of MLAs. In 1992, the Chief Scientific Officer asked the Institute to lead a review of the logbook prior to publication of a second edition. Eventually, the Institute took over responsibility for producing and issuing the logbook.

For those employed in the NHS, restructuring of the grades and the introduction of MLAs was not the only issue to cause concern. Long delays between completion of the Management Advisory Service (MAS) report *Review of pathology services' staffing and management* and its publication also had an unsettling effect on members in the NHS.

The Institute's response to the report was generally positive, with the mains points being: i) a multi-specialty district pathology service run by a medical director responsible for the overall provision of services, and a laboratory manager responsible for the analytical phase of the service; ii) a new grade of 'Technologist' who would staff the analytical phase and, with the pathologist, be involved in setting the objectives and standards for the service; iii) the introduction of the post of 'Medical Laboratory Analyst' who would be trained to undertake basic technical tasks; iv) while it recognised the role of the scientist in research and development, MAS considered that scientists should be remunerated as technologists and that local health authorities should determine the number of R&D posts appropriate to the service they provided.

The DH was not entirely supportive of the report. It had "doubts over the appropriateness of the MAS concept of a laboratory manager covering all specialties. The director of pathology may, however, require the assistance of an MLSO of appropriate grade in managing common services on his behalf". The DH obviously didn't realise that Principal MLSOs were already undertaking this task, and there were female pathologists! The Institute agreed that the three groups of staff proposed – pathologists, technologists and medical laboratory analysts – were appropriate for the needs of the laboratory. It also agreed that technologists should be engaged in setting the standards and objectives. It strongly endorsed the MAS conclusion that local employers should determine the number of technologists employed as scientists and suggested that it might be more appropriate if they were employed on short-term contracts for specific purposes. The DH did not comment on the amalgamation of scientists and MLSOs into a single 'Technologists' group, but said it preferred to await the outcome of discussions taking place under the chairmanship of Professor Roger Dyson, adding that if there were any proposals for change these would have to be negotiated through the appropriate Whitley Council. However, judging by the rather acrimonious reply to a letter sent to the Institute from the DH and by a letter from the Chief Scientific Officer, Dr F P Woodford, in February 1990, the recommendation was not likely to find favour.

After a series of meetings of representatives of the IMLS, ACB, RCPath and ACP, the Dyson Committee produced a consultative paper on a possible integrated structure for non-medical staff in pathology. This was published in *The Gazette* in July 1989 and sent to the DH. The paper was considered by Council in September 1989. Although it had reservations about some aspects of the proposal, it agreed with the broad thrust of the paper. However, no action was taken on the proposals and, despite the fact that biomedical science has become an all-graduate profession with a high proportion of the membership holding higher degrees and Chartered Scientist status, the division between the two groups of staff remains to this day.

Who should manage pathology was not a new issue, as the ramifications from the 'Fife dispute' were still being felt nearly a decade after its conclusion. Great disappointment and anger was felt by the profession when the DH issued the circular EL (89)P/17. This set out new guidelines for the management of pathology services. However, the guidelines were not new as the circular merely reiterated and reconfirmed the guidance given in 1974 in HSC (IS) 16. Given the comments on the Management Advisory Service report *Review of pathology services' staffing and management*, this was not surprising. The new circular made it clear that a department would be managed by a medical consultant who would report to the Director of Pathology. It further stated that: "We therefore do not advocate the concept of a 'Laboratory Manager' responsible for the work of technical staff in all specialties and reporting direct to the Director of Pathology". The Institute wrote to the DH to express its profound disappointment in the circular. In the view of the Institute, it was "incredible that in spite of the MAS recommendations and the government White Paper *Working for Patients*, which endorses the Griffith management philosophy, the DH does not realise that management should be undertaken by the 'most capable person'". The letter went on to point out that "the laboratory service has undergone enormous scientific and managerial changes which have not been recognised in the guidelines; these merely perpetuate an inefficient system. Some health authorities have already implemented practices which make these guidelines redundant". Sadly, these comments were generally ignored by the DH, although in reality the introduction of 'General Management' into the NHS in many ways superseded the guidelines.

***

During 1992 the Institute received advice on the lease it held for its offices at 12 Queen Anne Street (QAS) and it was decided that it would be financially advantageous to look for new premises and to sublet QAS. Although the lease had a further 25 years to run, its value would reduce significantly after the 20-year term had been reached. A detailed appraisal of the options was proposed, including relocation outside London; however, a move outside London was rejected for a number of reasons: ease of travel; London properties were no longer significantly more expensive than other cities; many of the organisations with which QAS interacted were based in London; and QAS staff were not considered to be 'mobile'. At that time the property market was depressed but there was evidence that it was reviving. The

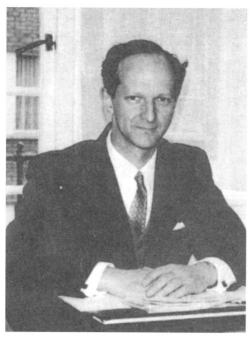

John K Fawcett

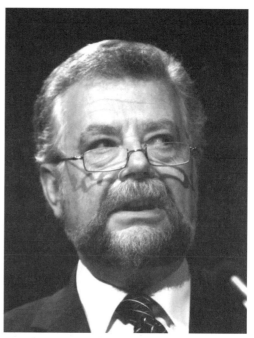

Alan Potter

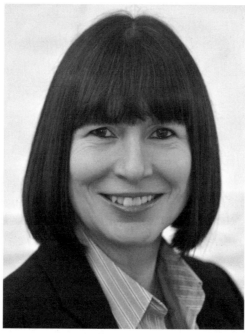

Jill Rodney

Institute had hoped to purchase a property with sufficient space to hold workshops/seminars for 125 people, but this was not considered to be a financially viable objective.

After looking at a large number of buildings, and changing property advisors, attention focused on a newly built development, 12 Coldbath Square, London EC1 5HL. A space planning exercise indicated that approximately 65 people could be accommodated legally in a lecture-style format in an area that could also act as a Council Chamber, and be divided to allow two simultaneous meetings. There was also sufficient space on the three other floors to accommodate the administrative activities of the Institute. Although initially valued at approximately £1 million for the 150-year lease, the price had been reduced. Council was advised that this was an exceptional price and extremely good value and it was agreed to proceed with the purchase.

To facilitate the purchase, a trading company, Institute of Medical Laboratory Sciences (Professional Services), was formed. The premises were eventually purchased at a cost of £477,000 on 18 October 1993. During 1995 the lease for 12 Queen Anne Street was disposed of, which greatly improved the finances of the Institute for that year.

Transfer to the new premises started at the end of 1993 and became the official address of the Institute on 1 January 1994. This date also marked a further change in name, from IMLS to the Institute of Biomedical Science (IBMS). When proposing the special resolution to the 1993 AGM, the President, David Browning, said that "The new name would reflect more accurately the Institute's broad membership base and enable it to widen its field of influence and recruitment. The new name would remove the perception that the Institute was confined solely to MLSOs in the NHS and the implication that it supported the widely unpopular title Medical Laboratory Scientific Officer". The report of the AGM shows that: "The resolution was passed, to great acclaim from the members present".

The offices and conference facilities at Coldbath Square underwent further refurbishment and modernisation in 2006, and in June 2008 the freehold of the building was purchased for £23,500.

***

Over 75% of the Institute's income was from membership subscriptions, with the remainder coming from examination and CPD fees, Congress and profit on investments. With a falling, or at best static, membership and increasing costs, the Development Plan recognised that there needed to be an improved approach to income generation. Several potential income streams were identified. Increasing the number of members was seen as the most beneficial form of income generation, and studies were established to discover what members and lapsed members saw as the advantages and disadvantages of belonging to the Institute. Recruitment initiatives that proved successful were the 'Member gets Member' campaign, the free student membership scheme, and a discount for those members who paid their fees on time. Student membership was extended in 1996 to include third-year IBMS-accredited BSc (Hons) students on laboratory placements and to full-time students on IBMS-accredited MSc courses. Both initiatives proved to be very successful and nearly 60% of the student members progressed to conventional membership.

A new non-corporate membership class of Affiliate was aimed at those working in medical laboratories and related fields but not training towards or qualified for corporate membership. At the beginning of 1993 there were 78 in this class of membership, and numbers rose gradually to stand at a little over 150 at the end of the century, rising to just over 200 in 2006.

As a result, total membership increased but this was boosted by the influx of student members. The number of Associates and Fellows remained more or less static (12,500–13,000) until 2004 when their combined total rose to almost 14,000, and to close to 15,550 the following year; the first year since the beginning of 1988 that the total exceeded 15,000.

***

Seminars and short courses not only provided support and advice to members and potentially non-members but also the potential for income generation. Providing these courses in cooperation with commercial course organisers had the dual benefit of providing income and prestige, with minimal practical input from the Institute.

Senior laboratory staff needed to acquire new skills. The development of a 'business environment' and increased scrutiny meant that the demand for meetings on these and related topics was increasing. Over the next few years the Institute provided national and local meetings on topics such as marketing, costing, workload measurement, accreditation, COSSH, workload indicators, SOPs, job descriptions and benchmarking. For those unable to attend the meetings, articles and reports on these subjects were published in *The Gazette*.

***

Between December 1997 and June 1998 there were five meetings of the IBMS/RCPath 'think tank' and these led to what was described in the Leader in the January 1999 issue of *Biomedical Scientist* as a "dramatic proposal". What was proposed was the merger of the IBMS and RCPath to form The Royal College of Pathology. The rationale behind the proposed merger was to bring the three professional groups, medical, clinical scientists and MLSOs, involved in pathology into one body, and was set out in a report entitled *Future self-regulation and representation of professional staff in pathology: A new Faculty for the College?* sent to members of both bodies at the end of 1998. The 'think tank' members and authors of the report were IBMS President Jocelyn Germain, Ivor Holiday and Alan Potter, and College Chairman John Lilleyman and five other members.

The plan was to set up a unified organisation, to regulate the competence of all professional staff involved in pathology, to set professional standards and represent all aspects of pathology in discussions with government and other external bodies. Their reasons for this were set out in Section 2 of the report: "For the last few years pressures to alter the configuration of diagnostic and academic pathology have gathered apace. Laboratories have been subjected to the need for accreditation, the threat of market testing and a push towards centralisation of services into bigger and more automated units. At the same time the medical and allied professions have never been more vigorously called to account by government and the media. Difficulties in the cervical cytology screening programme have repeatedly grabbed the headlines and poor professional performance will clearly not be tolerated in the health services in future.

"It is thus an extraordinary time for those working in laboratories in terms of adapting to change, defining and maintaining professional quality standards and making themselves heard in political circles. Because, however, the individuals concerned are represented by different professional organisations, there is potential for conflicting opinions from these bodies which is at best self-cancelling and at worst allows public argument between supposed colleagues collectively working for the good of patients."

The report pointed out that at one time the three groups were easily distinguished, as were their entry qualifications, training and roles, but the previously sharply drawn boundaries between them had blurred. While clinical scientists in consultant-level posts had quite different responsibilities from MLSOs, and as graduate entry to MLSO training was universal and as many obtained higher degrees, there was confusion about the relative responsibilities of non-consultant grade clinical scientists and more senior MLSOs.

The report suggested that the external pressures referred to had occasionally produced political tensions between the three professional staff groups and that this was particularly evident at times when the government sought to review the organisation of pathology services. It believed that public discord had probably been counterproductive for pathology and must be regarded as illogical and unnecessary. It felt that a single professional association to represent the whole of pathology was needed and that such an organisation would be a force for any government to reckon with and would have a real grip on professional standards and self-regulation. A Royal College of Pathology was proposed.

Reaction within the Institute's membership to the proposals was polarised, being either total support or total disagreement. In the words of a short report in the February 1999 issue of *Biomedical Scientist* "there is an aura of excitement developing on the subject". The report stated that many members had written with forthright views on the possible merger and they represented all shades of opinion. It was planned to prepare an informal synopsis of the letters for consideration at a meeting of the two bodies and, after consultation, "a detailed scheme may then be prepared for an annual general meeting or extraordinary general meeting". Unfortunately, none of the letters were available to us for consultation, nor were any published in the *Biomedical Scientist;* however, in view of the decision made at the March 1999 Council meeting, it can be assumed that there was a great deal of antagonism to the proposals from members of both bodies. The report in the *Biomedical Scientist* from the Council meeting read: "The think tank on IBMS/RCPath closer cooperation had now considered the reaction from both bodies and revised its proposals". In the *Annual Report 1999* it was stated that the original proposal of a merger between the two bodies was regarded as generally not acceptable, but it was agreed to create a general forum, possible entitled 'The Pathology Forum' to consider accreditation, competence and other issues. The following year saw this established as the Pathology Alliance, the founder members of which were the Institute, RCPath and the Association of Clinical Scientists. This continues to meet to discuss items of mutual interest.

***

Towards the end of the 1990s, NHS recruitment of suitably qualified trainees and the retention of qualified staff became extremely difficult. Government pay restraint policies and the exclusion of laboratory staff from the NHS Pay Review Body meant that salaries were around 30% behind those for other health service staff, and public service pay. In 1999 the starting salary for a graduate trainee MLSO was £7495, while a grade D nurse entered the profession on £14,400. In addition, comparative salaries in the private sector were generally much higher than those in the public services.

Many laboratories resorted to expensive locums to fill the vacancies, not all of whom were properly qualified, or used unqualified trainees and MLAs instead. This encouraged staff to leave and become locums, often to be re-employed in their original laboratories, which exacerbated the situation. Although the Institute was not a trades union, this did not prevent it from holding and expressing its views on the employment conditions of its members when these had a deleterious impact on the quality of the profession and the service it delivered. Indeed, since the birth of the NHS in 1948, three members of Council had attended the Whitley Council in an advisory capacity.

The IBMS Council developed a strategy to raise the awareness of the public, politicians and other opinion-formers, of the role of the profession, the difficulties it was experiencing, and the implications this had for patient care. It appointed a political lobbying company and a public relations company to advise it on this strategy. By the end of 1999 the PR company reported that over 10 broadcasts and articles had been used by the media. However, some opportunities had been lost as spokesmen or detailed information was not available. Unfortunately, due to a lack of corroborating data, the BBC Radio 4 programme *File on Four* had not used the Institute's significant input.

It was agreed that a survey to gather national statistics on staffing problems should be commissioned. The results of the survey, in reality, merely put numbers to what was already known and confirmed that there were major problems. Around 62% of respondents reported that they were below full establishment, of the trusts that sought to appoint MLSOs in 1999, 54% failed to fill all vacancies, and 18% failed in their attempts to appoint any new staff. In trusts seeking MLSO1s, 93% felt that the number and quality of applicants were inadequate, and 50% failed to appoint altogether. The turnover rate for MLSO1s was over 16%, and 61% of these cited low pay as their reason for leaving, while 19% cited stressful working conditions. A similar survey undertaken by the trades union MSF confirmed the results obtained by the IBMS.

There was intense media interest in the survey. The first story was published in *The Observer* on 23 January 2000. The following day, Alan Potter gave 24 interviews in three hours. Altogether, two news agencies, 45 national and regional newspapers in England, Scotland and Wales published the story, as did the news programmes on all major UK radio and television channels. Not surprisingly the subject then entered the political arena. Lord Hunt, a junior health minister dismissed the news as "long on allegation and short on facts" and denied that unqualified staff were being used. However, the DH acknowledged that there were staff shortages and that it would be "working with the IBMS to develop a solution to the career structure and salary problem to resolve this critical problem". Questions were asked in the House of Commons by Dr Vince Cable and other MPs.

Another part of the strategy involved a brief session for MPs at the House of Commons, which focused on the problems of the profession. To demonstrate the type of work carried out, blood cholesterol tests were offered to those attending. Many local branches and laboratories lobbied their local MPs and arranged for them to visit laboratories.

The outcome of this campaign was a salary award, effective from April 2001, negotiated by the trades union representatives on Whitley Council, which aimed to address the recruitment and retention problems. Employers were also reminded that they had, in the case of new appointees, the discretion to appoint to any point on the pay scale and that they could make local pay supplements of 20–30% to address proven problems.

Although there continued to be annual cost-of-living increases, the inequalities in the starting salaries for graduates in the NHS were not resolved until the implementation of *Agenda for Change* on 1 April 2007, when the starting salary became £19,166 per annum.

***

The Institute has recorded many 'firsts' in its history but it took 85 years from its formation, and 75 years from the admittance of Miss G S Brown as the first female PBLAA member, to the inauguration of Ms Jocelyn Germain as the first, and so far the only, female President of the Institute in 1997; a professional body whose membership in 2011 is now predominantly female.

Jocelyn Patricia Germain commenced her career in the Lewisham Group Laboratories in 1963, before transferring to the Institute of Psychiatry, rising to the grade of Senior 1 Technician. After a spell in the Department of Morbid Anatomy, The Hospital for Sick Children, Great Ormond Street, she spent three years as a Research Technician in the Department of Pathology at Guy's Hospital Medical School. In 1975, Jocelyn moved to the Royal College of Surgeons' Department of Dental Science, and then was appointed to the post of Chief MLSO and then Senior Chief MLSO in Oral Pathology at St

Bartholomew's and The Royal London School of Medicine and Dentistry. Jocelyn became a Fellow in 1971 and in 1975 was awarded the degree of Master of Philosophy from the Faculty of Medicine, University of London.

Jocelyn was an experienced teacher, lecturer and examiner in her specialty of histopathology, both for HNC and Fellowship, as well as teaching on the MSc course in Experimental Oral Pathology. In 1986 she became a member of the Histopathology SAC. The following year, she was elected a national member of Council and sat on a number of committees as well as being a member of the IBMS Accreditation Panel for BSc and MSc courses in biomedical science, and a member of the CPD Unit.

On becoming President Elect in 1996, Jocelyn took on the chairmanship of both the Operations and Education and Professional Standards committees, and also chaired the 1997 and 1999 Congress committees. During her time as President she sat on a number of important NHS and other committees concerned with the development, education and training of scientific and technical staff in the NHS including MLAs, as well as a CPSM working party on clinical scientists and MLSOs. She played a leading role in forging closer links with the RCPath, particularly as chairman of the Pathology 2000 conference committee. She was also active in CPA as both a member of the CPA Board and as a laboratory inspector from 1993. In 2002, Jocelyn was elected an IBMS Vice President and in July 2011 became a member of the Institute's History Committee.

***

By 1995 the PSM Act was, after 35 years, starting to show its age, and the Institute, together with the other professions covered by the legislation, participated in a review. The following year firm proposals to replace the PSM Act were published by the DH. The Institute's Chief Executive, Alan Potter, was appointed to the Bill Advisory Group, which was to produce the framework on which the new Act could be drafted. The draft Bill was completed towards the end of 1997. From the beginning it was clear that some of the requirements of the new Act would have long-term consequences for both Institute and profession. The first of these was the expected requirement for

CPD, and the Institute already had a well-established but voluntary CPD scheme. Higher education establishments had already begun to ask the Institute for advice on meeting these new requirements.

Although the *Health Professions Bill* was ready by the end of 1997, Parliamentary time was not available for debate, and it was not until 2002 that a mechanism popularly known as the 'Henry VIII procedure' was employed. Using this, clauses were added to the Health Bill which was under consideration by Parliament at the time, giving the Secretary of State for Health powers to replace the PSM Act, to abolish or amend existing statutes, and introduce new regulations relating to all health statutory regulatory bodies.

On 1 April 2002 the Health Professionals Council (HPC) became the registration authority. The Institute was represented on the shadow HPC Council by Neil Willis and Gordon Sutehall, the latter being a member of the IBMS Council. The HPC continued to operate CPSM rules until 31 March 2003, while undertaking a consultation on future arrangements.

It soon became apparent that a conflict of interest would exist if the HPC set standards of competence to practise and awarded certificates of competence. After discussions between the Institute, health ministers, the NHS Executive, the HPC and HUCBMS, in June 2002 the Privy Council granted the Institute the role of Awarding Authority. This meant that the IBMS would have the right and responsibility to assess the professional competence of MLSOs who wished to become registered with the HPC, and issue them with a Certificate of Competence. It took over this role on 1 July 2002, and on 1 April 2003 it was also given the authority to assess overseas applicants on behalf of the HPC.

It had previously been the responsibility of CPSM to issue logbooks, arrange oral examinations, and assess training laboratories and academic establishments. These responsibilities were taken over by the Institute, which set up a State Registration Unit at Coldbath Square to handle this additional work and issue certificates to those who had completed the competence assessment satisfactorily.

This additional activity, together with the increase in CPD, rising numbers of members and membership enquiries, the proliferation of postgraduate qualifications offered by the Institute, the award of Chartered Scientist status, and support for related organisations such as the Association of Anatomical Pathology Technology, the British Society for Clinical Cytology, the National Association of Phlebotomists and the Association of Medical Laboratory Assistants, placed considerable pressure on office space and staff. Therefore, additional premises were sought, and fortunately 5 Coldbath Square became available. The lease was purchased in June 2004 for £628,625, with the freehold obtained in February 2009 for £23,000. Additional staff were recruited and by 2005 the total number of staff employed by the Institute had risen from 24 WTE in 2000 to 34 in 2005.

Increased political scrutiny of pathology and other healthcare-related sciences led to the Institute becoming further involved with related professional bodies. The Institute took a leading role when the Federation for Healthcare Science (FHS) was formed in 2002, and it provided both the secretariat and Registered Office for the FHS. It was formed to act as an umbrella organisation to represent the interests of, and act as a single voice for, the 40 or so groups of healthcare scientists in the NHS. Among its aims are to enhance the profile of healthcare science and those professions working within it and to emphasise the roles performed relating to patient care, quality, clinical governance and health improvement – aims totally compatible with the objectives set out by the founders of the PBLAA in 1912. However, the Institute was already working closely with many organisations in the same sphere. The *Annual Report 2003* listed six organisations with which it was involved; however, reading elsewhere in the report and other publications it is evident that the number is under-recorded. In 2004 the number of organisations listed as the Institute's main partners had risen to 15, plus the DH and various working groups, committees and programmes set up with other organisations or government. By 2010 the number had risen to 17, plus a plethora of other committees, which placed even more pressure on staff, the executives, Council members and other representatives.

One aspect of the HPC consultation concerned protected titles. The Institute had long argued that the 'official' title under the PSM Act, Medical Laboratory Technician, and the employment title, Medical Laboratory

Scientific Officer, were both incorrect, outmoded and should be replaced by the more appropriate Biomedical Scientist. Unfortunately, Medical Laboratory Technician was enshrined in the PSM legislation and could not be changed without further legislation. The new Act provided the opportunity to rectify this anomaly. The Institute's evidence to the HPC consultation pressed the case for Biomedical Scientist as the protected title. However, other bodies were believed to advocate 'Medical Laboratory Scientist' as the title. In the event, only Biomedical Scientist was recommended to the Privy Council by the HPC, and, on 1 September 2004, this became the officially registered and legally protected title.

***

During 2007, Council started to make plans for events and ways to mark the Institute's centenary in 2012, and, to facilitate this, established a steering group under the chairmanship Mr David J Ricketts to consider how the occasion could be celebrated. Several events were planned including a float in the Lord Mayor's Show and a collaborative event with the RCPath, which would be marking its 50th anniversary in the same year. David also suggested that a book should be commissioned to update that written by Derek Farr. Regions and branches were also to be encouraged to mark the occasion and soundings were made with the Science Museum to gauge the extent to which the museum was prepared to mark the occasion.

***

No account of this period would be complete without recording the immense role played by Alan Potter in shaping the events that transformed what was, when he was appointed as Chief Executive, an organisation in decline, into a highly respected, vibrant and influential one. He brought considerable knowledge of the Institute, the profession and the health service to the post.

Alan Robert Potter MBE MPhil DSc(Hon) CSci FIBMS, started his career as a Student Technician in the Department of Pathology at Dorchester County Hospital in 1965. He trained in all disciplines, passed the Intermediate Examination, and then qualified in histopathology. In 1970 he moved to the Royal County Hospital, Winchester, where, after obtaining his Fellowship by

Special Examination in cellular pathology, was promoted to Chief MLSO. In 1976 he moved to the Royal United Hospital, Bath, as Senior Chief MLSO. While in this post he developed an interest in immunocytochemistry, and published several papers and wrote a chapter on the topic for the textbook *Clinical Cytotechnology*, lectured at polytechnics in Bristol and Portsmouth, and at Llandaff Technical College, South Wales, as well as acting as a cellular pathology examiner. In 1982 he completed a Master of Philosophy degree in the Faculty of Medicine, Southampton University, by thesis entitled *The Dating of Skin Wounds.*

He left Winchester in 1984 to become Principal MLSO at the Princess Margaret Hospital, Swindon, and later became an Assistant General Manager with responsibility for hospital support services and a coordinating role for paramedical services. In addition, he was project manager overseeing construction of the £15 million extension to the hospital, obtained a Certificate in Health Economics and was chairman of the Wiltshire branch of the Institute.

His role as Chief Executive was to guide Council and to ensure that its decisions were implemented, but anyone who holds such a post for 21 years will, by virtue of experience, have a great depth of knowledge to bring to any discussion. This, combined with his skilful diplomacy and engagement with politicians and other influential opinion-formers made him a formidable ambassador for the Institute, and he played a major role in developing the current high standing of the IBMS and its members.

Most of the events that occurred during Alan's time in post have been covered elsewhere in this account; however, it is worth reiterating them: change of Institute name; purchase of 12 and 5 Coldbath Square, and their refurbishment; replacement of the Triennial with Congress; establishment of relevant BSc and MSc degrees, and of an IBMS accreditation system; establishment of CPD scheme and the rebirth of Institute professional qualifications; establishment of Institute Certificate of Competence for registration purposes; Deputy Registrar, Registration Authority; Member and then Trustee of The Science Council; award of Chartered Scientist licence; formation of HUCBMS and the College of Biomedical Science; close working with the RCPath and other professional bodies; outsourcing of Institute publications and launch of website and online facilities; change of Institute membership structure; and establishment of Biomedical Scientist as the protected title.

In 2008, Alan was made an MBE "For Services to Science". A retirement dinner was held in his honour on 3 March 2011. The IBMS President, Kenny Rae, in his speech, remarked that Alan had started his career in Dorchester and ended it in The Dorchester. The President also pointed out that, during his term of office, Alan had worked with 10 Presidents, five Treasurers, and three DH Chief Scientific Officers, had attended 82 Council meetings and written 243 Leading Articles for *'The Gazette'*, as well as representing the Institute during visits to 19 countries. At the dinner, Alan was presented with the Sims Woodhead Medal in recognition of his immense service to the Institute, and he was elected a Vice President at the 2011 AGM.

The importance Alan Potter attached to the Institute's history was crystallised in a Leading Article he penned for *The Biomedical Scientist* in November 2010, in which he wrote: "I take the responsibility of the Institute to record and preserve the history of biomedical science very seriously indeed. If you lose history it can never be recovered". It was further emphasised when he commissioned this book.

In 2011, Alan was replaced as IBMS Chief Executive by Ms Jill Rodney, a pharmacist by profession and a former NHS trust chief executive.

***

The first decade of the 21st century has been perhaps one of the most turbulent and intense periods of the Institute's history. Major initiatives came thick and fast. The long-term impact of many of the issues and initiatives on the Institute, its members and the wider profession of biomedical science remain unclear. Some appear to have strengthened the role and status of the Institute and the profession at large; others may well have the opposite effect. If our treatment of these issues appears rather superficial it is because of this lack of clarity. It will need the vision of hindsight to more clearly unravel the impact of what are, in reality, more current affairs than history, and it is, after

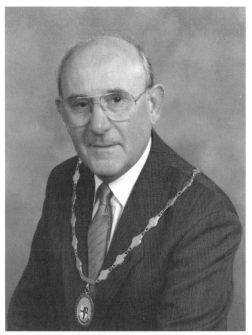

David M Browning

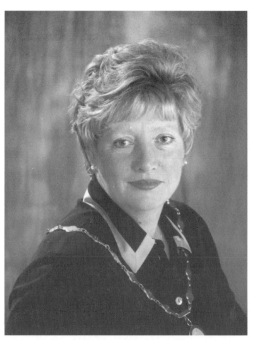

Jocelyn P Germain

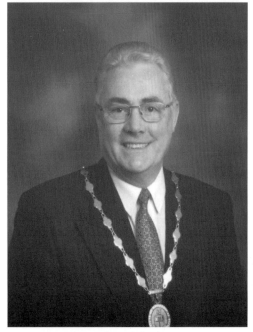

Martin Nicholson

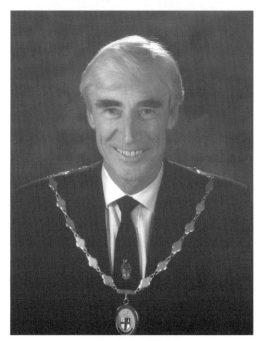

Russell T Allison

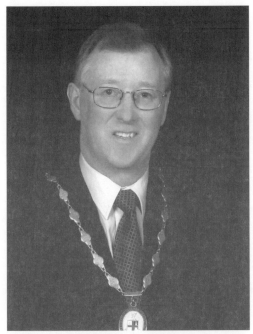

Edward M Welsh

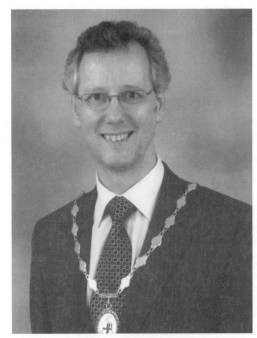

Gordon M Sutehall

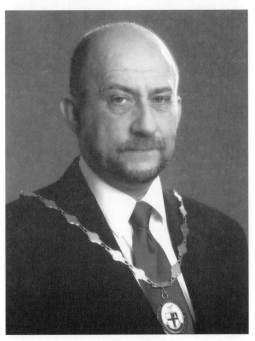

John R Stevens

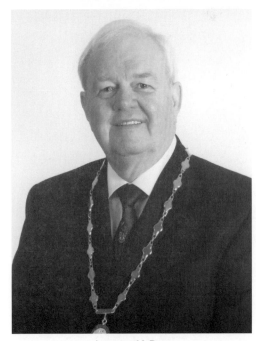

James K Rae

all, the role of historians to recount history not report current affairs.

The ramifications of *Modernising Pathology Services*, published in February 2004, the *Review of NHS Pathology Services in England,* chaired by Lord Carter of Coles, the second part of which appeared in 2007, and *Modernising Scientific Careers* will not be known for some time and it may take many years before they are completely understood. There can be no doubt, however, that the Institute will continue to be actively involved in the negotiations surrounding the implementation of these initiatives, to ensure that the standards of the profession are protected, maintained and advanced, as it has for the past 100 years.

Chapter 17

Epilogue

The Time Machine, a science fiction novella by H G Wells, was published in 1895, just a matter of months before John McLean made a tentative attempt to garner support for a laboratory assistants' association. In both instances, what followed is 'history'. Wells' work has spawned feature films, television versions and comic book adaptations, and has stimulated the minds of eminent scientists over the past century. Likewise, McLean's idea ultimately germinated and he and his laboratory colleagues were to see professional success that found application worldwide, as this account has sought to illuminate. To some extent, this history has been an exercise in time travel; what remains unavailable, perhaps impossible, is to journey forward in time, so the following conclusions represent an educated guess.

If the founders of the Institute were able to visit a 21st-century pathology laboratory they would, perhaps initially, find very little that they could recognise. Once they got over the size and complexity of the service and notwithstanding the automation, computerisation and digital communication systems, however, they would discover that there are techniques that have stood the test of time which would be familiar to them, such as the Gram and haematoxylin and eosin (H&E) staining methods, bacteriological culture techniques using Petri dishes, and section cutting using a microtome. They would also discover that principles on which their professional body, the PBLAA, was founded have also endured and, like the science on which the modern pathology service is based, have developed and expanded to meet the needs of the modern biomedical scientist.

As the range of techniques, analytes, equipment, microorganisms and therapies has expanded and increased in complexity, so has the Institute's involvement in education, training, examinations and the setting of professional standards, alongside the knowledge and skill of the those working in laboratories. They would also realise that the principles on which the PBLAA was founded – "To form a means of communication amongst the assistants; to supply information regarding appointments and to assist in the general advancement of its members" – remains at the heart of the IBMS. They may, now and in the future, be expressed in different words and in the mission statement style of the period, but there is no doubt that these principles will continue to form the basis on which the Institute functions in the future – the Institute's motto, *Disce ut proficias* (Learn, that you may improve), has enduring application.

***

How the Institute will develop, and whether or not it will still be in existence in another 100 years, is an intriguing unknown and it is not the role of the historian to speculate about the future; we may be allowed to operate the retrospectroscope but not the crystal ball. Nevertheless, as there are so many new initiatives and recent developments that potentially will bring about significant changes to pathology and the way it is practised in the UK, it will be fascinating to see how it responds to these on behalf of its membership and the profession at large.

Currently, the IBMS is a strong and thriving body with a membership of more than 20,000, it has good communications and relations with government and its agencies, as well as with related professional and educational bodies. The part it plays in the accreditation of qualifications and laboratories, its role in issuing certificates of competence for registration with the Health Professions Council, together with its CPD and postgraduate qualifications makes it a very influential organisation. By virtue of its membership, however, the IBMS is NHS-orientated and this is both its strength and potential weakness.

The different approaches to the organisation of healthcare in England, Northern Ireland, Scotland and Wales, and particularly the proposed devolution of healthcare management to the local level, Quality, Innovation, Productivity and Prevention (QIPP), local GP commissioning consortia, the centralisation and potential privatisation of pathology services, and real-term cuts in NHS funding could all have an adverse effect on this influence. The effect of the Carter Report and *Modernising Scientific Careers* has yet to be seen. In addition the amalgamation of laboratories, the expansion of automation, the rapid introduction of new technologies and the breakdown of the boundaries between disciplines all have the potential to reduce the number of qualified biomedical scientists needed in pathology.

***

As a result of analysing the past, it is clearly apparent that the current membership is less inclined to express opinions and views than was the case even 25 years ago. This is difficult to comprehend as there are certainly as many contentious issues to debate and modern forms of communication allow the instantaneous transmission of views. Perhaps a stimulus for greater communication is needed that would strengthen the Institute by closer involvement of its members. The Institute is potentially very vulnerable to economic pressures. Many of those who attend courses and conferences, such as the Biomedical Science Congress, depend on employers granting study leave and providing the funds needed; spending on postgraduate training and education is to a great extent at the discretion of the employer. In times of financial restraint, this type of spending may well be restricted, attendance at these events could fall and as a consequence prove difficult for them to continue in their current form.

The work of Council and the IBMS advisory panels also depends on the goodwill of employers to release individuals and on the other demands placed on members in their place of employment. Without this goodwill, much of the management of the Institute would become difficult, and alternatives to round-the-table meetings during working hours may have to be sought. Whether this will result in the greater use of modern communications technology or more use made of weekend meetings, as was the case in the early days of the PBLAA and IMLT, is not clear. One suspects that neither will be popular, but it is likely that persuading hard-pressed members to take on voluntary posts in branch, regional and national committees will become more difficult.

***

To ensure its relevance in the future, the IBMS may well have to look beyond its current constituency and traditional areas of influence to see how it can meet the needs and aspirations of related services, and perhaps expand into areas not covered by its current remit. This may well involve new classes of membership and other professional groups in the scientific community – it is, after all, the Institute of Biomedical Science, not biomedical scientists. Many of the current threats are probably short-term and subject to the will and whim of politicians and other influential groups, and will, no doubt, change over time.

What will not change, however, are the continuing advances in technology and the understanding of the underlying processes of disease, their diagnosis and treatment. What also will not change is the continued dedication of biomedical scientists to acquire the new skills and knowledge needed to provide an essential service to patients, and there is no doubt that the Institute will continue to serve and support its membership, as it and its predecessors have over the past century. However, whatever future role the Institute designs for itself, it is essential that it keeps an accurate and secure record of its activities and organisation to enable future historians to document and analyse its achievements.

APPENDICES

RULES OF THE PATHOLOGICAL AND BACTERIOLOGICAL LABORATORY ASSISTANTS' ASSOCIATION

1 Association shall be called "The Pathological and Bacteriological Laboratory Assistants' Association"

2 The objects of the Association shall be:

(i) To form a means of communication amongst the Assistants.

(ii) To supply information regarding appointments.

(iii) To assist in the general advancement of its members.

3 The Association shall consist of:

(a) Ordinary Members. Anyone holding the position of Laboratory Assistant in a Pathological or Bacteriological Laboratory or Museum who is 20 years of age and who has had three years' training shall be eligible for election as an ordinary member.

(b) Junior Members. Assistants under twenty years of age are eligible for election as Junior Members; on fulfilling the conditions specified in rule 3a, Junior Members become subject to the rules governing ordinary members.

(c) Honorary Members. Members of the Medical Profession who are intimately connected with the sciences of Pathology and Bacteriology can be invited by the Committee to become Honorary Members, and are eligible for election as President. The number of such Honorary Members shall be limited to twelve.

4 The Annual Subscription, due on January lst, shall be – Ordinary Members 5/ -, and Junior Members 2/6.

5 Every candidate for election must be proposed by two ordinary members who shall have personal knowledge of the candidate. The candidate and his proposers shall fill in the application form of the Association and forward the same to the Hon. Secretary and Treasurer, who shall publish the names in the Journal. If no objection to the candidate's election be lodged with the Secretary and Treasurer within twenty-one days of the publication of the Journal, the Committee shall proceed to elect the candidate. Should there be any objection to the candidate's election, the

Committee shall have full power to refuse the candidate's admission to the Association.

6 The government of the Association shall be vested in the office-bearers, who shall be elected from among the members, and shall hold office for one year but shall be eligible for re-election. They shall consist of *President, Vice President, Hon. Secretary and Treasurer*, and committee of five representing the following divisions: *Division A*, London and District, 2 representatives; *Division B*, Cambridge, Oxford, Birmingham, Bristol, Cardiff and Norwich, 1 representative; *Division C*, Manchester, Liverpool, Sheffield, Leeds, and Newcastle-upon-Tyne, 1 representative; *Division D*, Scotland and Ireland, 1 representative.

7 The President, Vice-President, and Hon. Secretary and Treasurer, shall be elected by ballot of all the Ordinary Members. The votes for the ensuing year to be counted at the annual meeting of the Committee.

8 The representative members of Committee shall also act as Divisional Secretaries and shall be elected by ballot of their respective divisions. Two umpires shall be appointed in each division to count the votes, and shall forward the result to the Hon. Secretary and Treasurer.

9 The Committee shall hold an annual meeting when the Hon. Secretary and Treasurer shall render a statement of his accounts with the Annual Balance Sheet.

10 The Hon. Secretary and Treasurer shall attend all committee meetings and general meetings of the Association, take minutes of the proceedings and discharge such duties as the Committee may direct. He shall further keep account of all receipts and payments and render such statement to the Committee as they may require. He shall also prepare an annual balance sheet for circulation amongst the members.

11 Any member whose subscription is one year in arrears will be considered to have forfeited his right to membership, and after due notice being given, the Committee shall have power to erase his name from the list of members.

12 If it be represented to the Committee that any member has been guilty of a misdemeanour calculated to discredit the Association, the Committee

shall have power to consider such report, and after hearing the defence of such member, if a majority of three-fourths agree, they may call on the member implicated for his resignation.

13 Any alteration of the rules of the Association must be passed by a three-fourths' majority of the ordinary members, the Hon. Secretary and Treasurer to have two months' notice previous to the Annual Meeting of the Committee of such proposed alterations or additions to the rules.

14 The Monthly Journal of the Association shall be issued by the Committee, who shall appoint annually an Editorial Sub-Committee of three, one member of the Sub-Committee to be the Editor.

RESULTS OF THE FIRST CERTIFICATE EXAMINATION IN 1921

Subject	Entrants	Passed	%
Pathological Technique	24	14	58
Bacteriological Technique	34	28	82
Museum Technique	17	11	65
Total	75	53	7
Special subjects	8	8	100

CLASSES OF MEMBERSHIP OF THE INSTITUTE OF MEDICAL LABORATORY TECHNOLOGY AT ITS FORMATION IN 1943, AND THE QUALIFICATIONS AND EXPERIENCED REQUIRED

Class	Qualification	Experience
Student	Preparing for Part I examination	
Ordinary member	Passed Part I examination	Three years
Associate member (AIMLT)	Passed Part II examination	Further two years
Fellow (FIMLT)	Passed two Part II examinations or one Part II examination plus a special subject	Further two years

SENIOR OFFICIALS OF THE PBLAA, IMLT, IMLS and IBMS

PRESIDENTS

PBLAA

1913	Professor J Lorrain Smith
1916	Professor Sir German Sims Woodhead
1922	Professor A E Boycott
1925	Professor H R Dean
1928	Professor W W C Topley
1931	Dr J A Murray
1934	Professor J McIntosh
1938	Professor J H Dible

IMLT

1942	Professor J H Dible
1949	Professor L P Garrod
1953	Professor R Cruickshank
1956	Professor E T Spooner
1960	Professor H A Magnus
1964	Professor A C Lendrum
1968	Professor G W A Dick

IMLS

1975	F J Baker
1979	D B Slade
1982	G Smart
1985	R G Fewell MBE
1988	E J Cloke
1991	A J Barrow MBE TD

IBMS

1994	D M Browning
1997	Jocelyn P Germain
2000	M Nicholson
2002	R T Allison

2004	E M Welsh
2006	G M Sutehall
2008	J R Stevens
2010	J K Rae

CHAIRMEN
IMLT

1942	C E Layng
1944	A Norman
1958	R J Bromfield
1961	W H Valentine
1964	G C Pascoe
1967	T S Lansley
1970	W H Finch
1973	F J Baker

VICE PRESIDENTS
PBLAA

1912–1915	R Muir
1916–1920	J McLean
1921	W A Mitchell
1922	H W Smith
1923–1924	F R Chopping
1924–1925	T D Hamilton
1925–1926	J W Manby
1926–1927	F E Soper
1927–1928	W A Mitchell
1928–1929	H P Hudson
1929–1930	W J Muggleton
1930–1931	C W Ashton
1931–1932	S J Denyer
1932–1933	H W Boot
1933–1936	A Norman

| 1936–1938 | A B Cheyne |
| 1939–1941 | C E Layng |

IMLT/IMLS

1942	J McLean
1942	A Norman
1943	F R Chopping
1945	S J Denyer
1958	R J Bromfield
1960	W H Valentine
1966	G C Pascoe
1968	G McKee
1969	L A Willis
1970	R J Lavington
1971	R Harper
1978	W H Finch
1981	F J Baker
1983	W R Ivory-Hollingsworth
1984	D B Slade
1989	J K Fawcett
1992	T S Lansley OBE
1992	R G Fewell

IBMS

1995	E J Cloke
	A D Farr
	G Smart
1998	A J Barrow MBE
	I R Holliday
2002	Jocelyn P Germain
	D Kilshaw
2003	M Nicholson
2007	E M Welsh
2009	G M Sutehall

GENERAL SECRETARIES

PBLAA

1912–1914	A Norman
1915	W J Muggleton
1916–1922	A Norman
1923–1927	H P Hudson
1927–1936	H Gooding
1936–1942	S J Denyer

IMLT

1942–1943	S J Denyer
1944–1946	J M Signy
1947–1970	R J Lavington
1970–1975	J K Fawcett

IMLS

1975–1988	J K Fawcett

CHIEF EXECUTIVES

IMLS

1988–1989	H M Lodge
1990	H Tate (Acting)
1991–1993	A R Potter

IBMS

1994–2011	A R Potter
2011–	J Rodney

TREASURERS

PBLAA

1912–1920	A Norman
1921	F E Windley
1922–1925	F E Soper
1925–1931	H W Boot

1931–1936	F E Windley
1937–1942	F A Croxon

IMLT

1943	R Hodgson
1944–1945	No separate treasurer
1946–1956	H A Barker
1957–1972	L A Willis

IMLT/IMLS

1973–1978	W H Finch
1979–1983	R G Fewell
1984–1989	A J Barrow
1990–1999	I R Holliday
2000–2004	G M Sutehall
2005–2008	J K Rae
2009–	J V Johnson

TRIENNIAL CONFERENCE DETAILS

	Triennial Conference year, venue and significant events		Keynote address/ Albert Norman Memorial Lecture
1952	London	Lectures held in LSHTM. Trade show on Wednesday afternoon at the Royal Free Hospital	Patricia Hornsby-Smith - Parliamentary Secretary to the Ministry of Health
1955	Nottingham	Produced draft constitution for International Association of Medical Laboratory Technologists	Dr G E Godber – Joint Deputy Chief Medical Officer – Ministry of Health
1958	Bristol	Albert Norman retired as Chairman of Council	Sir John Charles – Chief Medical Officer – Ministry of Health
1960	Blackpool	First Weekend Study Course	Professor C L Oakley
1962	Edinburgh	Golden Jubilee. Trade show increased to four days. Evening symposium on the *Coulter Counter*	Professor R Cruikshank
1964	Harrogate	Second and last Weekend Study Course	Professor G Belyavin
1965	Cardiff	Sixty six Companies exhibited in the Trade Show	Professor A C Lendrum – IMLT President
1968	Belfast	The first afternoon session on Laboratory Management	First Albert Norman Lecture given by Professor J H Biggart *The stones on which we build*
1971	Aberdeen	Public symposium - *Chest and Heart Disease* - held jointly with the Chest and Heart Association	Albert Norman Lecture – Sir James Howie *The qualities of a good technician*
1974	Sheffield	Televised public symposium on cancer. An IMLT stand staffed by members of Council. Historical section of the Institute formed. Last IMLT Triennial	Sir George E Godber Albert Norman Lecture – Professor Sir Charles Stuart Harris *The influenza problem*

1977	Liverpool	First IMLS Triennial. First Conference presided over by a President who was not drawn from the medical profession – Mr Frank Baker OBE, a Fellow of the Institute. Plaque to commemorate the formation of PBLAA unveiled	Rt Hon David Ennals Albert Norman Lecture – Professor D J Wetherall *Genetic engineering*
1980	Bath	Poster presentations formed part of the programme for the first time	Patrick Jenkin - Secretary of State for Social Services Albert Norman Lecture – Professor H D Wright *A multidisciplinary approach to diagnostic pathology*
1983	Stirling	Institute's dye approval scheme launched	George Younger, Secretary of State for Scotland Albert Norman Lecture – Professor Sir Cyril Clarke *Congenital abnormalities – are they preventable?*
1986	Southampton	The number of participants reached to over 2000 for the first time	Professor A P M Lockwood, Chairman of the Biological Council Albert Norman Lecture – Professor R R A Coombs *Harnessing the red cell for immunoassays*
1989	Warwick University (Coventry)	The number of participants rose to nearly 2400	Albert Norman Lecture – Professor E D Williams *Pathology and the new biology*
1992	Liverpool	Last IMLS Triennial, and final Triennial meeting	Albert Norman Lecture – Professor I McGregor *Towards a vaccine for malaria*

BIOMEDICAL SCIENCE CONGRESS DETAILS

Date	Opening Address	Albert Norman Lecture
30 October – 3 November 1995	Dr P Bourdillon – on behalf of the Parliamentary Under-Secretary of State for Health	Professor C Berry *Risks, Health and the Environment*
23–25 September 1997	Baroness Jay Secretary of State for Health	Professor Dame R Hurle *Ethical Issues in Pathology*
21–23 September 1999	Baroness Hayman Under Secretary of State for Health	Dr R Richardson *Death, Destitution and the Anatomy Act*
25–27 September 2001	Professor M A Richards, National Cancer Director	Professor Gordon Graham *Genetics with Everything: How Far Can We Go?*
29 September – 1 October 2003	David Amos NHS Deputy Director of Human Resources	Professor A M Johnson *The Sexual Health of the Nation*
26–28 September 2005	Andrew Lansley MP Shadow Health Spokesman for the Conservative Party	Professor Sir John Lilleyman *How Safe and Sound is the NHS?*
24–26 September 2007	Lord Carter of Coles Review of Pathology Services in England	Professor P Morrison *Familial Breast and Colonic Cancer – from Bench to Bedside*
28–30 September 2009	Professor I Cumming	Professor A Bradley *Advances in Organ Transplantation and Associated Immunological Consequences*
26–28 September 2011		Alan Potter *Crime of the Century or Chance of a Lifetime?*

PRIZES, HONOURS AND AWARDS

The Institute has, over many years, established a series of awards and prizes which allow it to recognise, reward and honour members, and others, for outstanding achievement or service. The conditions pertaining to some of the awards have, inevitably, changed as circumstances have changed, but they remain loyal to the original intention of the prize. The more established and significant of the awards are described below

Sims Woodhead Medal

This is the most prestigious of the Institute's honours and awards. The first medal was awarded to Albert Norman in 1924; up to 2011 the medal has only been awarded to 25 individuals.

After the death of Professor German Sims Woodhead in 1921 it was felt that the PBLAA and its members should inaugurate a memorial scheme to perpetuate his memory in the Association. In response to an appeal to members, the sum of £170 19s 9d (£170 99p) was subscribed. Of this, £27 10s (£27 50p) was spent on the preparation of dies for the medal, 10s 6d (52p) on secretarial expenses, and the balance was invested. A portrait of Sims Woodhead by Mr Goodrich was used by the artist, Mr J Pinches, for the medal. Several drafts were produced which raised the final cost of the design of the medal to £20.

In response to suggestions from members, the scope of the Memorial as originally drafted was altered, and the award of the Sims Woodhead Medal (as distinct from the Prize) was made as an expression of the Association's esteem in commemorating outstanding service to the profession.

Holders of the Sims Woodhead Medal

1924	Albert Norman
1927	Professor J Lorrain Smith
1930	Professor A E Boycott
1930	W A Mitchell

1933	Dr J A Murray
1939	Professor J McIntosh
1939	F R Chopping
1948	H A Barker
1948	Professor H R Dean
1949	Professor J H Dible
1950	J McLean
1952	S J Denyer
1954	R J Bromfield
1956	Professor D F Cappell
1965	W H Valentine
1969	R J Lavington
1971	Professor A C Lendrum
1975	Professor G W A Dick
1977	T S Lansley OBE
1984	Dr A D Farr
1988	J K Fawcett
1991	G Smart
1996	J R Mercer
1999	R T Allison
2011	A R Potter MBE

Sims Woodhead Memorial Prize

This prize was first announced in 1924 to be awarded from time to time. It was open to registered and ordinary members, and was for an essay on a topic set by the Sims Woodhead Memorial Committee. The prize was first offered in 1927, the essay subject being 'The Ideals of a Laboratory Assistant', but none of the scripts submitted was thought to be worthy of the prize. From 1952 the prize was awarded to the candidate who, at their first attempt in the Intermediate examination, obtained the highest marks in the written section. It was not awarded in 1970, the final phasing-out year of the Intermediate examination. From 1971 the prize was given to an Ordinary or Student Member, not more than 20 years of age on 1 January in the year of entry, for the best essay on a specified aspect of medical laboratory sciences. The prize was discontinued in 1982.

President's Prize(s)

The prize was inaugurated in 1913 by Professor Lorrain Smith, the first President. The prize of three guineas (£3 15p) was offered for an account of a piece of work carried out by a member. The judges took into account originality and gave the prize for what they considered to be the most valuable contribution to *The Journal*.

The competition was suspended for the duration of the First World War and in 1921 the then President, Sir German Sims Woodhead, offered two prizes for essays; one for senior members, on laboratory organisation and administration, and one for juniors, who were asked to give an account of their work over the past 12 months, and what they thought they had learned.

Since 1995 the IBMS President's Prize is an annual award of £100, presented to one student graduating from each university offering an Institute-accredited BSc (Hons) degree in biomedical science. Each university or college awards the prize according to its own defined criteria to graduates who achieve high academic distinction. The student must be an Associate member of the Institute by the end of January in the final year of the degree.

Greenfield Memorial Prize

This prize was established in 1924 to commemorate the name of Professor W S Greenfield, as a result of an open subscription to which his widow donated generously. Until 1939, two prizes were awarded annually: a Senior and Junior Prize. The Senior Prize consisting of the annual interest on the capital of the subscribed fund, together with a Greenfield Medal in bronze. This prize was open to all PBLAA members who held Certificate A or B. It was offered for the best essay or paper on original work in pathology or bacteriology, and preferably on the laboratory aspects of these subjects.

The Junior Prize comprised a sum of about £10, provided by Mrs Greenfield, and a Greenfield Medal in bronze. It was open to all Junior members of the Association on the following conditions: "That the candidate shall not be over twenty-one years of age, and that he shall submit some practical work which he has himself prepared in the department in which he is employed. This work must be certified by the Head of Department, who shall also enclose a statement of the service, character, progress made, and reasons or recommending the candidate for the Greenfield Prize". The candidate could also send in certificates bearing on his general education.

After some lapse during the war, the award of a single Greenfield Prize was resumed in 1944. It was awarded annually to a Fellow or Associate of the Institute for the best paper embodying original work in a branch of medical laboratory sciences, preferably on practical aspects. The prize consisted of the Greenfield Medal in bronze and interest on investments in trustee securities.

In 1978, following difficulties experienced with the trustees of the Greenfield Memorial Prize Fund, who were not members of the Institute and had not fulfilled the terms of the trust, the Institute regretfully relinquished its interest in the Fund.

R J Lavington Prize

This prize was established in 1977 to commemorate the name of Richard James Lavington. It was awarded annually to the candidate who, at the first attempt, received the highest marks in the four written papers of the Special examination for Fellowship. When the Fellowship examination ended, the prize was then given for the best MSc project in an IBMS-accredited degree. Currently (2011), the R J Lavington medal, diploma and a cheque in the sum of £500 are awarded by the Institute to the candidate who secures the highest final mark across all disciplines, in a single sitting, in the IBMS Higher Specialist Diploma examinations.

Malcolm Breach Prize

This prize was inaugurated in 1979 and awarded to the candidate who, at the first attempt, obtained the highest marks in the Special examination for Fellowship in bacteriology. When the Fellowship examination ended, the prize was then given for the best MSc project in microbiology in an IBMS-accredited degree. It is now awarded to the candidate who secures the highest final mark in microbiology, in a single sitting, in the IBMS Higher Specialist Diploma examination.

Company Members' Prize

The Company Members' Prize was established in 2006 by the Institute and its Company Members in support of the Institute's qualifications and to recognise individual achievement of high standards. The prize is awarded annually to the candidate who, at first attempt, achieves the highest pass mark in each specialist subject of the Higher Specialist Examination.

Research Grants

IBMS Research Grants are awarded annually to members of the Institute to support original investigation and other suitable research work. The grants awarded are usually between £500 and £4500. A single grant of up to £2000 to support original investigation may be awarded annually to a member of the Institute employed outside the United Kingdom or the Republic of Ireland.

Membership Awards

Vice President

Originally, Vice Presidents were elected annually by and from the membership of PBLAA. As they presided at the annual meetings they were to all intents and purposes the chairmen of the Association. Since the formation of the IMLT, Vice Presidents are Fellows whose nomination has been approved by Council and are elected at an annual general meeting.

Life Membership and Honorary Membership

These are two of the most distinguished honours that may be bestowed on a member of the Institute. These awards are of equal merit and standing, as they confer similar rights, but differ only in the requirements and timing of the award.

Honorary Membership is awarded to those who have given long and valuable service to the Institute at local or branch level. Life Membership is awarded to those who have contributed outstanding service to the profession and its professional body. It is one of the highest honours that can be bestowed on a member of the Institute.

Honorary Member and Honorary Fellow

When the PBLAA was founded, prominent pathologists who supported and assisted the Association were invited to become Honorary Members. When the IMLT was formed in 1942 these became Honorary Fellows (members of allied professions intimately connected with pathology were eligible to be elected). At that time, the number of Honorary Fellows was limited to 5% of the total membership. These are now persons who have given outstanding support to the IBMS or the profession, who would not normally become a Fellow.

EDITORS OF THE 'JOURNAL'

"The Provisional Committee, having agreed that the objectives of the Association would be best attained through the medium of a 'Monthly Journal', consider it advisable to issue their report (of the meeting held on 6 January 1912 at which PBLAA was officially founded) as near as possible to the form of the 'Journal' they recommend". These are the first words written in the first Journal published in July 1912. The first edition of *The Laboratory Journal* (Volume 1, Number 1) was published the following year in March.

Up to and including 2011, the position of the Editor of the Journal has only been held by seven men. Each has contributed to the development of a journal of international repute. The first was Albert Norman in his capacity as Secretary. After two years the role of Editor was separated from that of Secretary and Norman remained as Editor until 1950. He retained his association with the Journal as one of the two assistant editors until 1953; a period of editorial association with the publication spanning 41 years.

R J Bromfield was Editor from 1950 to 1966. He had previously edited *The Bulletin* from 1934 until 1950, when it was superseded by *The Gazette*, and became assistant editor of *The Laboratory Journal* in 1946. He quickly established the journal as a quarterly publication (until 1950 it had not been published regularly) of high scientific and technical value. In an article of appreciation written on Bromfield's retirement as Editor, W H Valentine said: "It would be difficult to overstate the importance of Bromfield's contribution, through its publications, to the life of the Institute." Bromfield was awarded the Sims Woodhead Medal in 1954.

C H Collins became co-Editor in 1966 and Editor in 1967. He also had a long association with the journal as a regular contributor to the Abstracts section, which from 1954 he collated and edited. During his stewardship it not only changed its format and title, but also saw the introduction of new scientific units, symbols and nomenclature. Chris Collins, sometimes known as 'Mike', had wide scientific interests; he not only edited the journal but also contributed book reviews and abstracts, wrote two books, a thesis and several papers. Although his contribution to the Journal was important, Collins was perhaps better known as an expert, with an international reputation, on mycobacteria and laboratory safety. He was a prolific author and editor of books, scientific papers and articles on laboratory safety and mycobacteria.

Collins was succeeded by D G Cramp in 1972, who, because of increased research and teaching commitments, relinquished the post at the beginning of 1975. He was succeeded by A D Farr, who took over from Volume 32, Number 2.

Derek Farr's period of editorial association with the Journal was second only to that of Albert Norman. During his tenure he was Editor, Editor in Chief and finally Consulting Editor. He was highly regarded in his own field of transfusion science and wrote a number of books on the subject. Considerable changes in science and laboratory practice occurred while Farr was Editor and he ensured that the Journal reflected these developments, and by so doing further enhanced its reputation.

Derek was a prolific author and editor, writing *Learn, that you may improve: the History of the Institute of Medical Laboratory Technology* and *Science Writing for Beginners* as well as editing a *Dictionary of Medical Laboratory Science*. He also applied his skills to the subject of steam railways. In 1983 Dr A D Farr was awarded the Sims Woodhead Medal in recognition of his services to the Institute and the profession, and was made a Life Member the following year.

Unfortunately, due to ill health, Derek Farr had to retire as Editor in Chief, but retained his connection with the Journal as Consulting Editor. His duties as Editor were undertaken by the then Deputy Editor Professor David Rogers, who in turn became Editor in Chief in 1997.

Professor Rogers was followed by Brian Nation in 1995, who joined the Editorial Board of what had become the *British Journal of Biomedical Science*, and was appointed Deputy Editor the following year. When David Rogers resigned at the end of 1997, Brian Nation was appointed Editor in Chief. In 2001 he left the NHS to join Step Publishing, which took over production and publication of the Journal at the beginning of 2002, and thus he became the first full-time professional editor of the Journal. As he had been appointed Editor of the *Biomedical Scientist* in 2001, Brian became the first person to edit simultaneously the quarterly Journal and the monthly *Gazette*, as well *Pathology in Practice*.

Since 1913 the Journal has reflected the development of the profession, the Institute and the sciences of pathology. It has had five titles, four page sizes, eight cover designs and, if in-house publication is included, six publishers. Its editors have coped with, and introduced, many changes in printing and publishing technology; from the early days when handwritten papers were the norm, through typed scripts, to word processed and electronically submitted manuscripts, from black and white to full colour, and from moveable type to full digital editing and printing.

Title	Editor	Tenure
The Laboratory Journal	A Norman	1913–1950
	R J Bromfield	1950
The Journal of Medical Laboratory Technology	R J Broomfield	1951–1965
	R J Bromfield and C H Collins	1966
Medical Laboratory Technology	C H Collins	1967–1970
	C H Collins	1971
	D G Cramp	1972–1975
	A D Farr	1975
Medical Laboratory Sciences	A D Farr	1976–1992
British Journal of Biomedical Science	A D Farr	1993–1995
	D J Rogers	1996–1997
	B R Nation	1998 to date

CODE OF PROFESSIONAL CONDUCT

The Council adopted a Code of Professional Conduct at its meeting held in March 1982. It was stated that the code should be followed by all members of the Institute. Every member of the Institute shall always:

1 exercise his professional judgement, skill and care to the best of his ability
2 fulfil his professional role with integrity, refraining from its misuse to the detriment of patients, employers or professional colleagues
3 seek to safeguard patients and others, particularly in relation to health and safety
4 treat with discretion all confidential and other information requiring protection, and avoid disclosing to any unauthorised person the result of any investigation or any other information of a personal nature gained in the practice of his profession
5 act in good faith towards those with whom he stands in professional relationship and conduct himself so as to uphold the reputation of his profession
6 strive to maintain, improve and update his professional knowledge and skill
7 promote the study and development of medical laboratory science and the education and training of medical laboratory scientists.

UNSUCCESSFUL PROPOSAL FOR A ROYAL COLLEGE OF PATHOLOGY

The main College to consist of:

Fellows and Members: by examination, published work or other existing routes.

Council: 24 elected members including eight diplomates from the Faculty of Laboratory Science.

Officers: selected by Council, including a medical president and a diplomate Dean of the Faculty. The medical president would help the College retain its membership of the Academy of Medical Royal Colleges.

SACs: as existing with Council members *ex officio*.

In addition, a **Faculty of Laboratory Science** consisting of:

Diplomates

1   Medical or science graduates who had passed the Part 1 MRCPath, but not the Part 2.
2   Medical or science graduates with at least four years' full-time experience in a relevant laboratory specialty and a) a higher degree in a relevant subject, b) Fellowship of the IBMS (non-graduate Fellows to be admitted by a grandfather clause), c) senior graduates in neither category a) nor b) sponsored by two Fellows and considered on an *ad personam* basis by the Faculty Board.

Associates (corresponding members with no voting rights)

1   Medical or science graduates working in a recognised pathology specialty with at least two years' full time experience.
2   Medical or science graduates formally enrolled in higher specialist training leading to the Part 1 MRCPath.

Faculty administrative structure
Dean: elected by Council from among diplomats.
Board: the eight diplomates elected to Council.

EDUCATION STRATEGY

In April 2011 a new Biomedical Science Education Strategy was published. It set out three priorities:

1 To support the biomedical science workforce to be suitably knowledgeable and skilled so that it can advance and maintain high standards of professional practice in response to changing workforce and service needs.

2 To encourage all members and potential members to be fully engaged with continuing professional development and through education and training develop the competence of practitioners of biomedical science to deliver first-class services and enhance the experience of patients and other service users.

3 To work with Institute members, education providers and others to ensure the development and maintenance of high standards of education and training as well as teaching and research in biomedical science, both nationally and internationally.

This continues to develop the intention set out when the PBLAA was formed "To assist in the general advancement of its members" and demonstrates how apposite the motto *Disce ut proficias* (Learn, that you may improve) has proved to be.

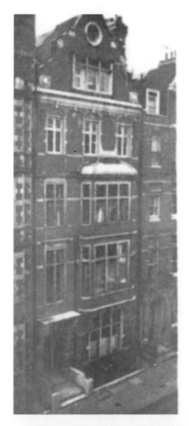

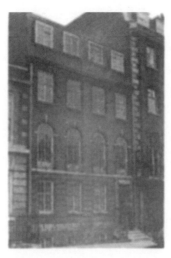

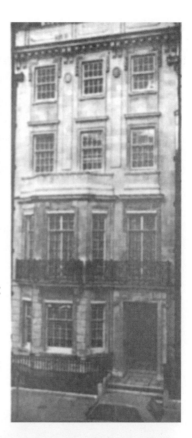

Previous Registered Offices:
from the left,
9 Harley Street,
74 New Cavendish Street
and 12 Queen Anne Street

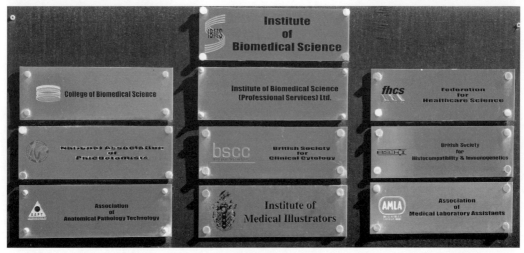

Name plates attached to the wall outside the current Registered Office at
12 Coldbath Square

INDEX